A STEP-BY-STEP FITNESS PROGRAM FOR A HEALTHIER LIFE

PRIME
MOVES

D1550993

A STEP-BY-STEP FITNESS PROGRAM FOR A HEALTHIER LIFE

PRIME MOVES

DIANE EDWARDS
with KATHY NASH

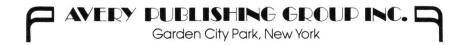

AVERY PUBLISHING GROUP INC.

Garden City Park, New York

The information and exercises presented in this book are based on the training, personal experience, and research of the author. Because each person and situation is unique, the publisher and author urge the reader to check with a qualified health professional before performing any exercise where there is any question to its appropriateness. It is a sign of wisdom, not cowardice, to seek a second or third opinion.

Cover Design: Ann Vestal
In-House Editor: Marie Caratozzolo
Original Artwork: Rachael Rodrigo, Widget Design, Mount Marion, New York
Typesetter: Widget Design, Mount Marion, New York

Special thanks to Connie Sciutto and James McBrearty, who served as models for the illustrations in this book.

Library of Congress Cataloging-in-Publication Data

Edwards, Diane.
      Prime moves: low impact exercises for the mature adult /
Diane Edwards with Kathy Nash.
        p. cm.
      Includes bibliographical references (p.) and index.
      ISBN 0-89529-394-3

      1. Exercise for the aged—United States. 2. Exercise therapy
for the aged—United States. 3. Physical fitness for the aged—United States. 4. Low impact aerobic
exercises—United States. I. Nash, Kathy. II. Title.

GV482.6E38 1992   92-12723
613.7'0446—dc20   CIP

Printed in the United States of America

10 9 8 7 6 5 4 3 2

Contents

For all my friends and students who have encouraged me to write this book. For my family, especially my husband, Lyle, for his patience.

Foreword

Can exercise programs offer any health benefits to older people? When mature adults want to improve their physical conditioning, can they expect any positive change? Twenty-five years ago, the prevailing medical opinion was that the older individual was "untrainable." The "experts" believed any physical conditioning that began after age forty produced only slight effects—and after age sixty, no observable improvement in function. Such was the "state of the art" as late as the mid 1960s, even though very little scientific evidence supported such contentions.

My colleagues and I at the Andrus Gerontology Center of the University of Southern California took a more optimistic view. In 1967, with support from the Administration on Aging, my colleague Dr. Gene Adams and I established a mobile laboratory in the Leisure World retirement community of Laguna Hills, California. We wanted to rigorously test the "untrainable" theory that was being applied to older adults.

For five years, we studied men and women whose ages ranged from fifty-six to eighty-seven. Our experiments tested the physiological response of the participants to exercise, measuring important factors such as oxygen transport, breathing function, cardiac output, and muscle function.

Our results clearly demonstrated that healthy older people who are involved in appropriate physical conditioning programs *do benefit.* In fact, an older person is not only retrainable but can benefit from physical exercise as much as or greater than—when improvement is translated into percentages—a younger person. Our results, which were criticized by some of our peers at the time, have been corroborated since, time and again, by investigators around the world.

Diane Edwards has an unusually fine background for encouraging anyone over fifty years old to exercise. She holds an undergraduate degree in physical education and a Master of Science degree in exercise physiology. This education is bolstered by her solid practical experience. For seventeen years, Diane has headed program development for Saddleback College at the Leisure World located in Laguna Hills, where she leads classes daily.

Her book is a welcome contribution to the current literature on aging. It should be helpful to both the older individual who wishes to remain healthy and the fitness instructors and program directors involved in exercise programs for seniors. Diane's approach works. The phenomenal growth of her Laguna Hills program—now probably the largest and most successful of its kind in the United States—is proof of this.

This book is extremely well-written in a lively style. *Prime Moves* makes interesting and stimulating reading. And it is my fond hope that more and more mature adults will realize the important contribution that exercise can make to their health and happiness.

Herbert A. deVries, Ph. D.
Professor Emeritus, Exercise Sciences
University of Southern California

Preface

Leisure World is a retirement community that fell into unexpected celebrity status after an important exercise study was conducted by Drs. Herbert deVries and Gene Adams. The study was the first of its kind . . . and the results were great news for anyone of any age who planned to grow older. Once the good news was out, Leisure World suddenly became inundated with requests from doctors, therapists, gerontologists, researchers, the curious, and mature adults of both sexes who wanted to be the best they could be. People wanted a chance to visit and even participate in the fitness program that had given new hope for the one thing that all of us do—age! The problem was that once the research was done and the four-year program was completed, Leisure World no longer offered a structured exercise program. Eventually, subsequent research was added to the original findings, but no immediate replacement program had been set up. With all of the requests, however, something had to be done. The officials at Leisure World decided to give an exercise program a try.

When the decision was made to set up an exercise program at Leisure World, it happened that our two young daughters had just started school and I was thinking about going back to work. I had learned that a position was open at the facility through a neighbor who worked at Leisure World. This seemed like the perfect opportunity for me.

I have always been fascinated with the miraculous inner working of the body, and interested in how the body grows, changes, and buffets its way through life. Not surprisingly, physical education was my college major. Contrary to what some might think, physical education is not a "cushy" major. I was required to take the same courses that pre-med students did—heavy doses of science, biology, physiology, and anatomy—and I loved it! For seven years I worked with junior high school and high school students. I modified my approach from the traditional notion of physical education classes to what I thought these classes should be. When I first started teaching, I saw a lot of "babysitting" going on during the time allotted for "gym." Students were playing games such as basketball, football, and soccer, but they weren't learning anything about their own bodies. I've always thought that physical education should include games and competition, but it should also teach students about themselves—their own inner workings. Teach them how to walk and run without injury; tell them which muscles are doing what; and even teach them how to control their weight and maintain lifelong health.

I was teaching physical education classes during the Kennedy years, when the students could try for the President's Council on Physical Fitness Award. It was an exciting time, a time when kids could push a bit and surprise themselves with results. I got the same rush of excitement when I taught swimming in Barstow, California. I got a lot of satisfaction watching kids go from non-swimmers to being able to swim the length of the pool.

When I became pregnant with our first child, I decided, in accordance with a game plan I had worked out with my husband, to quit teaching and stay at home. Two and one-half years later, our second daughter was born. I was delighted and busy with our little girls, but I always knew that once they started school I would resume the teaching I enjoyed so much.

After both girls were in elementary school, a neighbor casually mentioned that a position for an exercise director was open at Leisure World. The years at home hadn't changed my desire to help people know themselves a little better, and better themselves through the miracle of exercise. I decided to go for the interview. Dale Carnegie, the well-known motivator, would have been underwhelmed by that first exchange:

"Well, we don't think this is going to be successful, we're only doing it to satisfy a few people's whims," the interviewer grumbled. When he explained that the program would be part-time, I told him that the limited hours would be perfect for me. Since I had young girls, and this was my first return to work as a mom, being home for my children was a priority. I insisted that I be home by 2:00 p.m. when my girls returned from school. The interviewer agreed. Eager and ready to get back in the "exercise game," I began working on September 4, 1973. The Leisure World program was off to a slow, unimpressive start!

Shortly after that interview, I was shown to the area that was to be my work place. Known then as the crafts clubhouse, it was a small room divided in half—one section for woodworking, the other for ceramics. The wall between the two sections had been knocked down. Except for the dust and debris from the missing wall, the cement floor was bare.

My program experienced a low-budget start. I convinced the "powers that be" to cover the bare floor with indoor/outdoor carpeting. I had one exercise bike, one wall pulley, one mirror, a few folding chairs, and a card table for a desk. I had to obtain letters from the exercise and aging researchers at the University of Southern California and California State University at Fullerton to verify that—for safety reasons—I needed a phone in the room. My initial program was offered two days a week; my first several classes consisted of four men. Sometimes the men, sitting in chairs, did hand and feet exercises; other times, they used the equipment.

In the beginning, the program was a curiosity. But as people wandered by and watched the action, they must have figured we were up to something good, because attendance in my little groups grew. As interest and demand increased, we were able to buy more equipment—but not without a little bit of the old hassle I had experienced earlier.

At one point, I made a request for a blood pressure cuff (for monitoring blood pressure) and a stethoscope (used to listen to the heart). I felt this was important equipment to have around with any age group doing exercises, but my request was turned down. My superiors worried that the presence of this equipment would indicate that I was practicing medicine. Not a woman who is easily beaten, I waited for the next ordering period and jotted down a request for a *sphygmomanometer.* Sphygmomanometer is the fancy name for the same thing I had wanted before, a blood pressure cuff. This time I got it! Soon afterward, I was able to get the stethoscope, too.

Within a year, the Leisure World program grew to be much more than "the whims of a few people." I was logging more than a thousand repeat visits monthly for morning exercise enthusiasts alone in my small center. At this point I was given the okay to hire an assistant. In 1980, Leisure World built a half-million dollar facility to house our program. Today, two exercise physiologists and a staff of eight assist approximately 7,500 individuals who make 20,000 repeat visits monthly to our facility.

Shortly after I began at Leisure World, I did a little educational expanding myself. I went back to school and got a Master of Science degree in physical education, specializing in exercise physiology. An exercise physiologist looks at the *physical condition* of the body. Chronological age makes little difference to an exercise physiologist when considering a program for a client. For example, if there were two clients—both with diabetes—one forty years old and one seventy years old, both might be considered for the same exercise program. Body condition, not age in years, is the determining factor. Once I completed my master's program, I felt more ready than ever to plot the best course for the adults who wanted a better quality of life.

I love my work, and I know I can say that speaking for each one of the staff members at Leisure World. They have been hand-picked because they are excellent at what they do, and because they truly care about the adults who take the classes.

Some of the Leisure World staff is selected from local graduate students studying exercise physiology, As a forerunner in exercise for the mature adult, the Leisure World program has become an excellent training ground for the professional of tomorrow. The young men and women who participate in our Leisure World program and see the great results from exercise can pass the good work on—men and women who are sixty, seventy, eighty, and even ninety years old can expect and experience an independent, quality life. The key is to keep moving. *Use it or lose it!*

I attribute much of the success of this program to our quality staff. We don't run a "fling and flex" outfit at Leisure World. Our recommendations are based on scientific research and the physical condition of the participants. Customer satisfaction has helped us establish a good rapport with the medical community. Some doctors tell their patients, "Don't talk to me about exercise, go talk to Diane."

I know the first class that I described at the fitness center—the one with a few men sitting in chairs and wiggling their extremities—was underwhelming. But we have come a long way since those first few weeks. And what we're doing now is anything but old folks stuff.

Today, the Leisure World Fitness Center has thirty-six exercise bikes, eight treadmills, four rowing machines, four hand-crank bicycles, a hip-thigh machine, some shoulder-exercise equipment, wall pulleys, computerized bicycles and rowing machines, step machines, and weight-lifting equipment. And none of it is gathering dust! It is common to see people waiting to use their favorite machine.

Admittedly, it's impossible for me to climb inside your mind and see what you are visualizing when I discuss the Leisure World Fitness Center, but I'll bet in nine minds out of ten, the image is wrong. The exercise programs that are prescribed are very much like the ones that would be assigned to young people. The progression may be slower, but the work is much the same. Most who start our program are not quitters, and thanks to some hard work, we've got some pretty nice bodies at Leisure World.

We have some nicely defined chests that do justice to tank tops, and some lean torsos. Though muscular, slim bodies are nice, they are not our first priority. Our main concern is to get our participants into a healthy condition that allows them to live life fully and independently. Our weight machines can be adjusted to provide a wide range of resistance. Each workout, geared to the individual, includes arm, shoulder, and leg-strengthening exercises. Strong arms can carry groceries, and strong legs can support the body's weight, enhance balance, and make it a lot easier to get around.

Everyone in our program understands the importance of getting their bodies to work for them. This awareness influences the effort they put into the exercise classes. Step into our gymnasium for our strenuous General Conditioning class and you'll get fifty minutes of real exercise, not something watered-down to placate advanced age. We start moving—forward, backward, and sideways. Legs and knees are lifted high and with enough spirit and energy to keep time with a Sousa march. We work out to the pulsating beat of popular top-ten songs. We use that great 1-2-3-4 beat for leg lifts and for anything else that needs attention. And when we have had enough of that, we put on a tape of the charleston. The action is boop-oop-de-doo nonstop. That's how it goes. Even in between tapes, my class is moving, moving enough to seriously test the energy level of the college students who periodically stop by to see what's going on. Our General Conditioning class includes a strenuous twenty-minute low-impact aerobics workout, and there's definitely no rest time once we hit the mats. We do all the exercises that younger exercisers do: sit-ups, push-ups, leg extensions—the same movements recommended to battle bulge.

If this class is a little too much to begin with, participants can select a less-advanced workout such as the one done in the chair-exercise class, or they can take part in our walking, water exercise, and individualized exercise programs. Those who have had a serious illness or physical impairment don't have to forgo the effort to improve their conditioning—they simply have to take it a little slower.

Introduction

Do you drag yourself tiredly through your afternoons? Do you believe 7:00 p.m. is a reasonable bedtime? Is getting out of the bathtub becoming an Olympic challenge? Is it difficult to get into the back seat of a car and impossible to get out? Can you sleep anyplace, anytime—except in bed? Are things just "not the same"?

Unfortunately, for many, the answer to some of these questions is "yes." What used to be an active life, filled with get-up-and-go, has turned into a distant memory. Sadly, growing up for some has meant growing old or, even worse, growing "old and tired."

"Old" is difficult to define; I've seen twelve-year-olds drag themselves through the day as if they were a hundred, and I've seen great-grand-mothers enthusiastically peddling on bikes. "Tired," however, is as easy to spot as the wilt in the voice and the cloud of resignation hanging over the head. Anybody can get tired.

Personally, I believe in growing up, but I don't believe in that old and tired business. You'll never catch me describing someone as "over the hill" or "half-a-century old." I prefer to think that fifty-year-old-plus people have a half-a-century to go, that they've gotten all the kinks worked out, that they're mellowed like fine aged wine, and that the best is yet to come. Anyone fifty-plus has been through enough to make them inter-esting . . . and anyone who has been around longer is downright fascinat-ing! They can talk about a different time, a time when there were "good" girls and "bad" girls, handmade clothes, and home-cooked meals; about a time when the moon was something men and women wondered at instead of landed on.

In many ways age is great because it makes you so smart. Getting to mid-life isn't easy. Why, if you survived the same hoops and hurdles in a corporation that you've coped with in everyday life, they'd make you chairman of the board! Yes, you've come a long way—some of you further than others—but don't botch it by giving up now.

Eventually, all of us head into the sunset years. (I like sunsets. I love to watch that brilliant orange ball warm the quiet evening sky, so I don't mind comparing the aging process to sunsets.) So call this aging business whatever sounds good to you (something positive, please!); but while reflecting on times past, that identifying number that marks our stay on this planet, keep this in mind: high numbers don't mean the fun's done. The middle and older years should be a wonderful time in life, a time to take time out. Kiss the grandchildren. Hike. Travel. Visit. Take up mountain climbing if you must! At one time it was expected that wise men and women of a certain age would languish through their twilight years planted on a front porch or glued to a rocker in a corner of the living room. And there they were expected to wait out life with a little less animation than an art deco accent piece.

I have written this book to remind all of us that such ho-hum expectations of our older years are wrong. Life at any age can be active, fun, and filled with get-up-and-go. Exercise, like love, is not only for the young but also for the "not-so-young." Trust me, there's nothing wrong with, and everything right about, grandmother and granddad getting up, out, and on with it. If you're reading this from your armchair in the living room, it might sound a little crazy at first, but I can back up what I'm saying with nearly twenty years of research, testing, and work experience. Here's to the good life!

PART ONE

It's Never Too Late

Overview

Get ready to preserve and strengthen your body through proper exercise. I know that you are anxious to get started on your journey to the "new" you, but first, take some time and begin at the beginning. Part One of *Prime Moves* presents easy-to-read chapters that provide valuable information on exercise and its positive impact on the human body.

"The Exercise Experiment" presents positive physical results that can be attained through proper exercise. These results, taken from controlled study groups, are so encouraging that they serve as an incentive to anyone wanting to get involved in an exercise program. Chapter 2, entitled "Why Exercise?" discusses the positive impact that exercise has on such common conditions as high blood pressure, diabetes, and depression. Success stories are also included in this chapter. Chapter 3, "Getting Started," defines basic items that serve as goals when exercising: terms such as endurance, flexibility, range of motion, agility, and reaction time. Topics on proper dressing for the occasion are also presented in this chapter. The final chapter in Part One, "Designing Your Own Program," includes lists of suggested exercises geared for specific physical conditions as well as important keys for ensuring success.

Armed with determination and the spirit of adventure, prepare to get yourself into the best shape possible. Congratulations, you've just taken the first step in taking charge of your own good health!

CHAPTER 1
The Exercise Experiment

In 1967, Herbert deVries, Ph.D. and his associate, Gene Adams, Ph.D., received a government grant from the Administration on Aging to do research on exercise and the older person. deVries and Adams wanted answers to simple but important questions:

- If you had never exercised in your whole life, could you start exercising at age seventy or eighty?
- If you were a football player in high school but never exercised through your productive years (age twenty to fifty), could you start exercising again?
- Could exercise improve physical conditions such as blood pressure, resting heart rate, amount of body fat, and sleep patterns?

Drs. deVries and Adams also wanted to develop a safe, effective, scientific fitness program for older people. Exercise for the older adult was a novel idea twenty years ago, so the members of the group—researchers and volunteers—had their work cut out for them! deVries started his studies with male volunteers at the Leisure World retirement community in Laguna Hills, California. Leisure World established one of the first active senior-lifestyle retirement communities. Laguna Hills is nestled in the rolling hills of Southern California, so the beautiful scenery and mild temperatures provide the perfect place for getting out and about. It was the perfect setting for some action-packed testing.

The men's results were so encouraging that the women at Leisure World—not to be outdone by the men—campaigned to get themselves involved in the same program. They wanted to see what women could do when put to the same tests.

These initial studies spanned four years, but the good results have continued. The initial testing results showed that there could indeed be fitness and well-being for many mature adults. As a result, the lives, the way of thinking, and the physical well-being of many have been changed for the better.

For the exercise experiment, the researchers chose more than two hundred male and female volunteers, aged fifty-six to eighty-seven. Each volunteer underwent a thorough physical examination to confirm basic good health, but there were no prerequisites for fitness. Some of the participants had been active all of their lives and still played golf and tennis regularly; others hadn't exercised since their teens.

These experiments on exercise seemed to get everyone's heart started. Some participants in deVries' and Adams' program went above and beyond the sessions to also take part in programs offered through the Leisure World Recreation Department. Leisure World recreation offered swimming, golf, horseback riding, and shuffleboard. All volunteers were monitored by tests measuring body responses before, during, and after both the experimental and "just-for-the-fun-of-it" sessions.

Six weeks after the program started, the researchers could see dramatic changes in the participants. Blood pressure readings dropped; the percentage of body fat decreased; maximum oxygen capacity increased; arm strength improved; and electrical activity in the muscles (a sign of nervous tension) diminished. Most of the volunteers continued to improve, though at a slower rate, for eighteen to forty-two weeks, until they reached their peak levels of fitness.

Many participants reported added benefits: a woman plagued by headaches for years no longer needed daily doses of aspirin; her headaches disappeared. A man with chronic lower-back pain reported, "I no longer know I have a back." After two months of exercise, a volunteer who had been having continual problems with irregularity and constipation no longer had to rely on laxatives. Troublesome kinks in backs and joints vanished. Some people said they had never slept better. Several commented that they were now more sexually active than they had been in years. Even those people with mild illnesses improved.

Regular exercise seemed to turn back the clock for the volunteers. Men and women of sixty and seventy became as fit and energetic as those twenty to thirty years younger. And the ones who improved most were those who had previously been the least active and the most out of shape.

Walter, the oldest volunteer, was eighty-seven years old when he signed up. Walter's family, friends, and doctor had one objection: they feared that he was too old. So Walter was monitored even more carefully than the "mere" youngsters in their sixties and seventies. Walter not only completed the fitness program but remained active and healthy for years afterward. But Walter was only one example of the good news the experimental test results brought (deVries, 1974).

During the four years of Dr. deVries' exercise study, a long procession of adventurous senior volunteers took part. More often than not, the volunteers who had taken part in the program improved physically and mentally. That first program and those first volunteers proved an important fundamental point—it is never too late for fitness.

Other studies on exercise and the mature adult have followed the preliminary research done by Drs. deVries and Adams. And the original findings—that it is never too late for fitness—have been confirmed again and again. Men and women over fifty are just as capable of exercise and can get just as much benefit from it as the young and middle-aged. For older men and women, exercise has an extra payoff—it slows, stops, and even reverses some of the deterioration associated with aging. Older people who become and remain active may not be reborn, but they certainly are rejuvenated. Sounds too good to be true, doesn't it? How can something as simple as exercise have the effect of a fountain of youth?

Exercise increases the strength, endurance, and efficiency of the muscles of the heart, easing its workload. It appears to slow the closure of the blood vessels, and it may build up new networks of small blood vessels through the heart and body to transport oxygen more efficiently. Exercise improves breathing by increasing the capacity of the lungs to accept oxygen and strengthen the muscles that make the ribs expand and contract. It halts the loss of lean muscle and burns up excess fatty tissue. Exercise not only stops mineral loss from bones but also builds up the bone mass. For instance, joints that are arthritic due to osteoarthritis respond to appropriate, regular exercise. Studies now show that the right exercise, combined with estrogen replacement therapy and an increase in the daily intake of dairy products, does increase bone mass. It delays the impact of the aging process on reaction time and movement speed. And it works wonders for the mind as well as the body. Participants in the first and subsequent programs reported more energy, less tension, more restful sleep, and fewer feelings of depression (deVries, 1974). Certainly these good results are enough to encourage all of us to *use it or lose it.*

We don't promise instant miracles at Leisure World. No exercise program can! Nobody comes into one of my classes on crutches and walks out under his or her own steam within the first hour. But we do have a program that can ease forgotten muscles into shape, increase stamina, and steady one's balance. With these plusses going for you, you will become much more independent, ready to live life on your own terms. If you've got strength, flexibility, and endurance, you can help *yourself.*

Think of the things you need to do to remain independent. If you can't get out of bed due to stiffness, aches, and pains, your day is over before it has even begun. Even small tasks such as brushing your teeth, combing your hair, and tying your shoes require flexibility. Getting out of the bathtub without help requires leg strength. You need good balance for dressing and shoulder flexibility to be able to reach the zippers and buttons on the backs of garments. Buttons themselves can require a Herculean effort from an arthritic hand.

The fact is, to enjoy life, you need a well body. I want you to be able to do even simple tasks of daily life yourself. I want you to be able to carry your own groceries, or even better, to carry your own golf clubs. Remember, given a few tenacious genes, anybody can live long, but it takes a special person to live a long life with style! I'm betting that special person can be you.

CHAPTER 2
Why Exercise?

Exercise includes many kinds of activities and movements. *Recreational exercise* is meant for enjoyment and relaxation. *Therapeutic exercise* is meant for the correction or prevention of a particular problem. Sometimes an exercise can be both therapeutic and recreational. For instance, swimming the breast stroke, with careful attention to arm and shoulder movements, can meet both the recreational and therapeutic needs of someone with arthritis of the shoulder.

You see, there's a lot more to exercise than a little movement. There are many different types of exercise, and each has a specific purpose. A *range-of-motion* exercise helps maintain a joint's complete movement by moving a body part through its maximum available range of motion. It includes movements such as those experienced when extending and moving arms and legs in wide circular motions. These movements require some degree of flexibility, so I would recommend doing some flexibility exercises to loosen up a bit before trying any recommended exercises. This will reduce your chance of injury and improve your range of motion. A *strengthening* exercise helps a muscle's ability to contract and do work. Doing sit-ups is one way of strengthening abdominal muscles. *Endurance* or *aerobic* exercise improves the body's capacity to use fuel and oxygen. Swimming, bike riding, jogging, and brisk walking are aerobic pursuits. Some exercises, such as dancing, are designed to improve coordination. Other movements enhance balance and the ability of the whole body to work together. For instance, I often have people in my exercise classes stand on one foot for balance.

Some stand straight up on one foot with their other foot lifted off the floor; others stand on one foot, lean forward, and extend their dangling leg behind them. Whatever approach keeps them balancing on one foot is the best approach for them. Even if you start out wobbly, doing these movements regularly will improve your balance.

One exercise rarely achieves two goals. For instance, strengthening exercises will not significantly affect endurance, and range-of-motion activities will not necessarily improve strength. Total exercise programs must consider all goals and include activities specifically designed to achieve each of these goals.

Today, one of the most important goals of exercise is the relief of body aches and pains and even relief from what some call the "ravages of time." For a long time, people thought that once you contracted such health problems as arthritis, diabetes, or artery trouble, it would complicate the rest of your life. Now I'm not saying that exercise can make any of these complications go away, but it *can* do a lot to turn them into silent partners. This chapter looks at common body disorders that perplex and annoy both the young and the old; it shows how exercise can help lift the spirits, loosen the joints, and get you on the right track.

LONGEVITY

The main thrust of this book is to get you to exercise because it's good for you. "Good for you." How many times can you remember your mother using these words? Well, like your mom, I'm telling you that exercise falls into the "it's-good-for-you" category. By sharing real-life experiences and solid research I hope that I can show you why. With exercise you can experience top-notch living at any age.

But what about the premise that exercise can extend life? Who lives longest? How do you achieve a "quality" later life? Doctors, researchers, therapists, and ordinary folks are interested in the answers to these questions because nobody wants to spend his or her last years hooked up to a life-support system. So my colleagues and I have been particularly interested in learning if exercise could add zest and even years to life.

Dr. Roy Walford, a researcher at the University of California at Los Angeles Medical School, believes that discoveries in genetics and immunology will make it possible to slow down the aging process, increase average life expectancy to 120 years, and extend the maximum lifespan to 150.

"People who are seventy will look as if they are thirty-five," says Walford, "and people who are one hundred will only look fifty" (Walford,1983). If Dr. Walford is correct, our lives will change dramatically. Signs of better things to come can already be seen in the successes of some of my students.

Ruth and the Good Life

Ruth, from the Mayer clan of Metro-Goldwyn-Mayer fame, married a Hollywood director named Roy. Life around the movie industry meant a lot of entertaining that started with dinner and continued into the wee hours of the morning. And Roy and Ruth weren't known for letting any dust gather under their feet.

Barcelona, London, Naples, Tokyo, and Hong Kong are just a few places that this couple's life travels have taken them. The first thing Ruth did when she arrived in a new city was to take lessons in the language of that country. She felt it was a necessity for getting around. The next thing Ruth did was to get out and about and enjoy the wonderful places the new country had to offer.

A fifteen-year resident of London, she'll tell you that it's, by far, her favorite city. Maybe that's because she was lucky enough to have a reserved English friend who felt that all Americans need to be educated. The two made a perfect match. As tutor and tutee, the pair gallivanted all over England to historical sites and museums, Ruth has always looked at life as one adventure after another, and it has been especially fun, she admits, because of her husband's profession. Ruth and her husband have even attended parties (by special invitation) with Queen Elizabeth of England.

"Here I am, a person who has lived in Europe for twenty-three years. I did all the wrong things," she laughs, "and had a marvelous time." Ruth will confess that a lot of her eating during those gypsy years consisted of fried foods, gravies, and steaks, with lunch at three in the afternoon and dinner at midnight. Ruth also admits that the last thing she thought about during that time was exercise. There just wasn't time.

Ruth would have lived happily ever after in England if it hadn't been for her weak throat, which was irritated by the wet English weather. On a trip to the United States, Roy happened upon Leisure World in Laguna Hills, California. He was truly impressed. "I just love Leisure World, and you will love it," Roy told his wife. But Ruth had different ideas about the potential move. "I won't go there," she replied. "I'm a big-city girl and you're not going to put me way out there in the country." Ruth lost that argument but won a whole new, wonderful lifestyle in Southern California.

Ruth and Roy have been at Leisure World for seven years now. Ruth quickly discovered the classes and especially enjoyed the nutrition class. She loves to learn, so learning about the body and the proper way to nourish it was as much of an adventure for her as delving into British history, or wandering inside an art museum.

The last place anyone ever expected to see Ruth was in an exercise class. She'd always made it clear that she wasn't the exercise type. A small, fragile woman with dancing brown eyes and a properness that comes with years of taking tea with the English, she laughs easily and dots her conversation with words such as "marvelous" and "enchanting." And Ruth loves to laugh, but by her own admission, Ruth would never have taken on the physical adventure of exercise if she hadn't gained weight.

"I'm only five foot-one," she explains, "I can get fat quickly." Today, Ruth is far from fat. In fact, she's in great shape. At age eighty-six, Ruth walks two miles every morning and joins an exercise class three or four times a week. Her new exercise program has kept her body energized and her husband pleased. "The other day my husband said, 'Ruth you look pretty good; you got thin!'" she laughs. "And I *feel* better than ever!"

Milt: Conditioning an Unhealthy Body

When Milt was two years old, a bout with rheumatic fever kept him sickly and in bed until the age of eight. At one time during his illness, Milt's doctor predicted he would not live through the winter and advised Milt's parents to head west to California. They did, and Milt's health improved. He was able to live a normal existence.

The next years in California were glorious ones in Milt's life. He played like he'd never played before, participating in soccer, baseball, swimming, and anything else that allowed him to move. With his new life, Milt swore off medications. As far as he was concerned, the prescriptions hadn't worked before and he wasn't about to try them again.

As he grew, he approached every area of his life with great enthusiasm. A brilliant financier, Milt first worked as a comptroller for Saks Fifth Avenue. After a few years, he retired from Saks to work for another large corporation. These financially healthy years were, unfortunately, much less healthy for his body. "I worked seven days a week, twenty-four hours a day," he admits, "and, of course, there were lots of dinners and drinks. I was the first one in and the last one out of the office. I smoked three packs of cigarettes a day. Because of that habit, I slept sitting up and often had to breathe in a bag." This was Milt's lifestyle for nineteen years.

When Milt and his wife arrived at Leisure World, he was five feet seven and a half inches tall and weighed 165 pounds. Once at Leisure World, Milt humbly claims he took advantage of my knowledge. While that may be true, it's important to note that he did an awful lot to help himself. He got back into exercise with the zest of the kid who had come to California years earlier. Within months, the effort resulted in a streamlined, healthy Milt who, today, at seventy-six years old, weighs in at 135 pounds and does more in one day than some people do in three months.

As soon as he gets up, Milt does twenty minutes of exercise. This includes a combination of stretching exercises plus forty to seventy-five push-ups. After breakfast, he takes an hour-long bike ride before heading to the pool to swim thirty-six non-stop lengths. (That's a half-mile swim!) Milt also isn't afraid to take on that strenuous General Conditioning class (See Chapter 7).

To all this, Milt adds what he calls "social and mental gymnastics." He and his wife, Bess (his wife of fifty-four years who has joined him in the new, healthier lifestyle), entertain five or six nights a week. When they're not entertaining, both take advantage of courses offered at local schools. In his "spare" time, he volunteers his CPA talents to local organizations.

ARTHRITIS

Arthritis is one of the oldest diseases known. A painting done by the Neanderthals more than 40,000 years ago depicts an arthric man who is stooped and walks with bent knees. Arthritis occurs in all races and at all ages. Thanks to research and new insights, arthritis doesn't mean the end of the road.

Mary: Relieving Arthritis Through Exercise

Mary was a long-time sufferer of arthritis of the spine. "I used to wake up in the morning with my whole body aching," she explains. While waking up with arthritis was bad enough, arthritis complicated the rest of Mary's day as well. She couldn't reach for the paper on the walk in the morning; she couldn't bend for the dishes in the lower cupboards. Mary's doctor recommended that she take eight aspirins a day for the pain. When Mary complained that taking all of those aspirins might cause her stomach ulcer to flare up, the doctor recommended she also take an antacid. He also suggested that Mary move her dishes from the lower cupboard, where the stretch to reach them had proved painful, to the upper cupboards, where they were in easier reach.

Mary didn't take her doctor's advice because it didn't make sense to her. For a while, she was stuck with the pain of spinal arthritis and the pinched nerves that accompanied the ruptured discs in her spine. She did have surgery for the ruptured discs, but the loss of feeling on the outside of her left leg remained even after the operation.

In February of 1987, Mary and her husband, Russ, moved to Leisure World. But it wasn't until August that the exercise and nutrition classes caught her eye. Today, Mary has no trouble when reaching for dishes in the lower cupboard and even less trouble with a nagging spine. She's also eight and one-half pounds lighter than she was just a few months before.

"I think exercise is the key," she says, and exercise she does. She and her husband attend an exercise class four days a week, a weight-reduction class twice a week, and they follow a one-hour walking program three days a week (both want to make walking a six-day-a-week habit). It's easier now because they have the time, and it's more fun because of the support group a class situation gives. But best of all, it's great to be free of pain!

Was Mary's experience just a fluke? Not from what I'm seeing in my classes. Many of my students have experienced the pain and swelling that comes with arthritis, but selected exercises seem to calm the savage arthritis beast.

HIGH BLOOD PRESSURE

High blood pressure is a major risk factor in the development of artery disease, especially in the blood vessels to the heart and brain. Abnormally high blood pressure can be lowered with medication, but some side effects can occur. These side effects can range from headache, dry mouth, lethargy, and depression to an inflamed pancreas and even impotence. Any and all are good reasons to investigate alternatives to prescription medicine for controlling blood pressure. Not surprisingly, researchers have looked into exercise as a blood-pressure controller, and the findings have been good (Morehouse et al, 1971).

CORONARY ARTERY DISEASE

Consider the benefits of a well-conditioned heart. In one minute, with fifty to sixty beats, the heart of a well-conditioned person pumps the same amount of blood as the average person's heart pumps in seventy to seventy-five beats. Compared to the well-conditioned heart, the average heart pumps up to 36,000 more times per day, 13.1 million more times per year. That's a lot of unnecessary wear and tear.

Coronary artery disease is the major cause of heart disease and heart attacks in America; it develops when fatty deposits build up on the inner walls of the blood vessels feeding the heart. Eventually, one of the major coronary arteries may become blocked—either by the buildup of deposits or by a blood clot forming in the artery's narrow passageway. The result is a heart attack.

Lou and the Moment That Changed His Life

"I was walking in the neighborhood one morning, but I was having trouble even completing the first block, so I turned around and headed home. By the time I reached the porch, I could barely make it up the three steps to the door. As I grabbed the handle to the screen door, I was gasping for breath and clutching my chest. I collapsed in the hallway in serious need of medical attention."

Lou admits that he thought it would never happen to him, but those sharp pains were hard to ignore. The doctor told him he had *angina pectoris*, severe chest pains due to an insufficient supply of blood to the heart. Lou's EKG (electrocardiogram) resulted in an abnormal reading. A specialist was recommended.

Fearing surgery, Lou discussed alternative approaches with his doctor. An advocate of the natural approach to healing, Lou's doctor agreed to having Lou try a diet and exercise-treatment program. This "new way of life" requiring strong will and determination would have been a challenge for men half his age, but Lou was undaunted in his efforts. He also agreed with his doctor that if this non-surgical approach didn't work within a certain amount of time, he would make an appointment with a specialist.

It wasn't easy, especially in the beginning; Lou had to change a lifetime of habits. He had to pare his five-foot-eight-inch, 170-pound frame down to something more acceptable. "Sentenced" to a 1,200-calorie-a-day diet consisting mainly of vegetables, Lou admits it was a challenge.

He was a nervous wreck when he returned to the doctor's office for his first progress report, but his fears were put aside when the EKG showed a marked improvement. It wasn't long before Lou's doctor added exercise to his treatment. At the time, Lou couldn't even walk the length of this back-yard without having an angina attack, but eventually he improved. Walks in the yard progressed to walks around the block, then several blocks, and finally, to three miles a day. Imagine what an accomplishment that is for someone who couldn't walk a few feet just eight months before! Best of all, Lou's angina attacks became less frequent.

For his winter exercise program, Lou moved indoors with an exercise bike. He started by riding a mile, but by spring he was up to twelve miles a day. The next summer he was still following the strict diet, and he was biking or walking for exercise.

On the two-year anniversary of his program, Lou was taken off his old medication. For the first time in two years, he was able to drive a car.

In February 1983, nearly four years to the day that Lou had first visited his doctor for heart trouble, he was a different man; he was no longer the 170-pound heart-attack candidate who first rejected surgery. "You're do-ing so well," his doctor told him, "I'll tell you one thing—if you die anytime soon, it isn't going to be from a heart attack."

Today, Lou weighs 148 pounds, eats mostly fruits and vegetables, and watches his salt and sugar intake (occasionally treating himself to ice cream on Sundays). Exercise is a natural part of his daily lifestyle. Lou is sincerely grateful for the support given to him by his doctor, family, and friends, and for the quality of life he enjoys every day.

Lou had a wonderful experience, and I shared it with you so that you might know that there's hope at any age in any situation. I'm certainly not recommending that you throw away your prescription drugs and blindly follow a program such as Lou's, just be sure to consider all the alternatives when it comes to taking care of yourself.

DEPRESSION

Bad mood. I think we all know what that means. Like it or not, we've all experienced the emotional doldrums that can ruin the day. Your mood can shift many times during a twenty-four-hour period. Most moods are a reaction to what's going on in your life. If you've had "one of those days," you can feel happy, excited, outraged, sorrowful, and exhausted by it all by the time you hit the bed. Other moods are less fleeting, and may settle in like a bitter winter frost leaving you depressed or anxious for weeks on end.

For at least a decade, exercise has been recognized as a mood elevator. The quick mood fix of running, in particular, is one of the most researched experiences. Sports psychologists have even studied running as an antidote for clinical depression. The findings hold that working up a sweat is good for both the mind and the body.

Studies done by John Geist, Ph.D., and his co-workers at the University of Wisconsin Medical School conclude that a regular program of running is as effective as traditional psychotherapy in treating serious depression. And running is a great antidote to normal, everyday anxiety (Geist et al, 1979). In a series of studies done at the University of Wisconsin by William Morgan, Ed.D., one of this country's leading sport psychologists, the results proved positive. Participants who were worried, frustrated, or fearful were given anxiety tests. Then they ran. After running, the participants scored lower on anxiety tests (Morgan, 1979).

My experience has shown that not only running, but other forms of exercise, such as a good aerobic workout, a serious swim, a challenging bike ride, or a brisk walk, can be powerful antidotes to depression. Intense and prolonged movement works wonders for both the mind and the body.

For several years, researchers and runners have discussed *endorphin* levels. Endorphins, the body's naturally occurring opiates, are found to play a role in the so-called "runners high," or for the feeling of contentment that follows any serious workout.

This is a fact: something good happens when you exercise. Vigorous exercise, like fast walking, stimulates the body's production of these mood-influencing endorphins. They are the body's natural pain killers. They can produce the same effect as morphine, but they do not dull the mind—in fact, they may even increase mental alertness! These same natural chemicals may be responsible for reducing depression, improving the ability to handle stress, increasing the ability to relax, and creating a positive state of mental well-being (Lamb,1984).

Research has recently been conducted on the role of a hormone called *noradrenaline.* Noradrenaline is believed to be a mood enhancer. The presence of noradrenaline in runners and exercisers is higher than in non-runners, according to the work of Richard Diestbier, Ph.D., of the University of Nebraska (1986). Increase in the production of noradrenaline during running or other aerobic exercise may be what sends the "feel-good" message to the brain. Revving up the body's natural mood elevator seems a better way to treat depression than with artificial stimulants, as is often done.

Feeling good. Flying high. On cloud nine. Rejuvenated. Serene. Tranquil. Vigorous. No matter how it is said, one thing is clear: exercise is a natural high.

DIABETES

There are two main forms of diabetes: one strikes at any age and is due to the failure of the pancreas to produce insulin; the other, and more common form, develops during adulthood because with age the production of insulin lessens. Diabetes seems to run in families. Nearly a third of diabetics over forty years old have a family history of the disease, but abusive lifestyle (one that includes an excess of sugary and fatty foods and no exercise) can make you a prime target for this disease.

Diabetes strikes different people in different degrees. Some diabetics need insulin in the form of pills or injections, but diabetes that begins in middle or older age can often be controlled by diet and weight reduction alone.

Grace: Controlling Diabetes with Exercise

Grace was diagnosed as having diabetes in 1944, shortly after her daughter was born. At the time, research into diabetes was limited, so knowledge of the effective use of insulin was not as clear as it is today. For a while, both the doctor and this mother of five puzzled over what amount of insulin would be needed day to day, because the thirty-year-old mother's needs seemed unpredictable from moment to moment. Stress, diet, travel, holidays, and even the excitement surrounding the birth of a child could send her body into a tailspin. This could mean anything from mild confusion for the young mother to insulin shock, requiring trips to the emergency room at the nearby hospital.

At first, Grace depended on her doctor to come up with the magic insulin potion that would make her normal, but it wasn't long before she decided to try to take care of the problem herself. Grace chose exercise as the answer and she became a walker.

That was almost forty-five years ago. At the time, walking was considered an odd thing to do, so Grace became something of a neighborhood celebrity. On any given day, Grace could be seen sprinting with her youngsters trailing behind.

Her daily hikes worked. As long as she could walk, Grace could control, and even lower, her insulin intake. On days when these treks were cancelled due to ice and snow or postponed because of travel, Grace's feet would swell and she would have high blood-sugar readings on her urine tests. On these days she could be heard wistfully saying, "If only I could just get out and walk."

This woman's recognition of exercise in the control of her diabetes was right on target. Today's research backs up Grace's urge to get out and hit the road as a method to control her diabetes.

WHAT ABOUT YOU?

Before embarking on any exercise program, it is important to check with your doctor or health-care provider. Once you've gotten your doctor's approval, review the exercise programs I offer in this book. Consider your physical condition and your goals, then select the exercises that are best for you. Your program should include both endurance (aerobic) activities—rhythmical and continuous action such as walking, swimming, and biking—and general conditioning exercises geared toward improving specific areas of the body.

Let's say you're an avid walker and strut your stuff vigorously three days a week. That's a great aerobic workout, but for full conditioning you'll need to add some general conditioning exercises to your program. If you start with the first exercise in either the Sit-Down or the General Conditioning Workout (Chapter 6 and 7) and you work your way to the end of the section, you will have exercised your entire body. However, it is not necessary to complete all the exercises in either workout to reap the benefits.

You might not have time to go from start to finish, or you might be suffering a few aches and pains aggravated by some of the exercises in the program. Then do whatever you can. I've included suggested exercise programs—selected from the offerings in the book—for certain physical conditions. These are safe and they work.

Use it or lose it! I think that is the most important message I can give you. *Move.* It's never too late and you're never too old. Exercise is for everyone, and that includes the young at heart.

CHAPTER 3
Getting Started

For years, physical fitness only applied to athletes. Strength training was only for muscle builders; flexibility was only for those interested in dance and gymnastics; endurance training was for track and field athletes. The rest of us sat on the sidelines and watched. But things have changed. Physical fitness is not only for star quarterbacks and gold medal-winning athletes, it is also for regular people like you and me who have become health conscious.

I've talked a lot about what researchers, study groups, and successful exercisers have done, and there's certainly no shortage of good results. I'm hoping these good results will get you to rethink what you're doing for yourself and redefine the meaning of being physically fit as it applies to *your* body.

WHAT DOES IT MEAN TO BE PHYSICALLY FIT?

I intend to keep myself physically fit until the day I depart for that great gymnasium in the sky. My definition of a physically fit person is someone who has the energy, stamina, and strength to do what he wants to all day long, and still have enough left in reserve for emergencies. You don't have to be an Arnold Schwarzenegger or a Milt (page 14)—you simply need enough get-up-and-go to get things done that make *your* day. We're not signing you up for the Olympics, we're merely trying to sign you up for more "life" in your life.

Now, if my goal is to be an able, active, and independent person, I'll need certain physical characteristics such as endurance; flexibility; strength; balance; agility; coordination; full range of motion in my arms, legs, and torso; and a quick reaction time. This chapter takes a look at these aspects of physical fitness and gives you enough background to understand why I recommend certain exercises for particular conditions (see Chapter 4).

Endurance

If you have endurance, you have the ability to be physically active for an extended period of time. For instance, a person with endurance would have no trouble taking an hour-long walk. Endurance is affected by a number of things; heading the list is a body that is able and willing. An injured skeletal system could hamper extended exercise, and weakened connective tissue could stop you a few minutes into an effort.

A good exercise program, one that includes aerobic as well as general conditioning exercises, will condition the entire body so that there are no weak links. A conditioned person performs for a longer period of time and recovers from the extra effort quickly. A conditioned person has more energy and a greater working capacity, so that a daily task, such as carrying a suitcase or a bag full of groceries, will be no problem.

Flexibility

No matter what age we are, we all need flexibility—to zipper dresses, and to wash and scratch our own backs. Our flexibility (or lack of it) can actually determine what we do in life. Flexibility is important for doing fun things, like swinging a golf club or developing a mean backhand on the tennis court.

The average inactive adult loses approximately 4 percent of his flexibility every decade after age forty. The important word here is *inactive*, because active people in their eighties can be more flexible than an inactive thirty-year-old. The fact is, if you don't move your body and body parts, the body makes adjustments. Aging and inactivity can contribute to the actual shrinkage of our connective tissue. This body adjustment can limit motion and often results in pain and injury. Don't worry, there are exercises that can remedy this.

If you are past age forty, or haven't exercised in a while, I recommend what are called "static stretches." This means getting into a stretched position and holding it. For example, sit on the floor with your legs together and stretched straight out in front of you. With your arms outstretched, lean forward. Touch the farthest point on your legs without bending your knees! Do the best you can. Whether you're touching your knees, calves, ankles, or holding your toes isn't important. Static stretching is a very individual thing and not competitive. It is important that you use no bouncy or jerky movements while reaching forward. Once you've done your best stretch, hold that position for at least thirty seconds. This is a static stretch.

While sitting on the floor, legs outstretched, some people may choose to do a "ballistic stretch." This is a combination stretch and forward bouncing motion that alternately stretches and relaxes the muscles. Beware, however, that this movement can cause excess stress on the joints, especially if there has been joint degeneration or arthritis. Beginners or anyone with physical limitations would be better off doing static stretches. Both work, but either approach takes four to six weeks of regular stretching to increase flexibility.

It doesn't take long for the men and women in my exercise class to realize one thing—women are usually more flexible than men. No one is sure why, but men shouldn't be discouraged; they, too, will see improvement if they stay with it.

When you begin stretching, you may notice that one side of your body is more flexible than the other. We often use one side of our body more than the other and this tendency can contribute to back problems.

Try to stretch all parts of your body—shoulders, hips, and lower back. Don't forget your neck, hands, legs, and feet. Stretching is a good antidote for leg cramps. Just stretch the leg for thirty to sixty seconds and those nasty calf cramps will disappear (85 percent of the time). Some excellent stretches for countering leg cramps are provided in Chapter 8.

Strength

As we age, our bodies make adjustments, one of which is a change in total body muscle. From age twenty-five to age sixty-five, we lose about 20 percent of our muscle tissue. But the effect of this loss depends greatly on what the condition of the body was like when the muscle change began to creep in long, long ago.

People of all ages need muscular strength. I am not suggesting that everyone become a muscle-bound athlete, but I am saying that it does a body's mind and soul good to feel the independence that a good constitution can bring. There's nothing nicer than that little phrase, "I'll do it myself, thank you."

What kind of lifestyle did you have at age twenty-five? If you were physically active at work or in recreational activities, then you probably had a lot of muscle tissue. If you were the type of person that had a desk job and a sedentary lifestyle, you probably had less muscle tissue when you were younger. If you had a lot of muscle tissue to begin with, then losing 20 percent is no big deal; but if you didn't have much to begin with, then it could be a serious problem later in life. You can lose muscle bulk and flexibility and gain fat in its place.

In the front-center section of your body, between the the breastbone and the front of the pelvis, is a long vertical muscle called the rectus abdominus. This muscle can become shorter and weaker with age and inactivity. Its change not only affects the abdominal area but total posture as well. Without the strength of that center muscle, the shoulders and head move forward, creating a stooped-over position.

Do you know that your head weighs approximately twenty pounds? To get an idea of how heavy this is, pick up a bowling ball that weighs between thirteen and fifteen pounds. Now think of that twenty-pound weight perched on the top of your neck. This weight, coupled with the force of gravity and ineffective abdominal muscles, can cause all sorts of problems. It can put a strain on the small bones in the upper back (especially when arthritis or osteoporosis is present). A weakened rectus abdominus muscle that has been covered with fat (commonly known as "midriff bulge") can put stress on the lower back. This weakened muscle can no longer hold the abdominal organs in their proper place, which can put a squeeze on the digestive system since the rearranged stomach and intestines cannot work efficiently. But exercise can improve the strength and flexibility of all the muscles concerned—abdominal, upper and lower back, chest and shoulders. Remember, that stooped-over posture that is associated with old age is more often the result of poor physical fitness, particularly the loss of flexibility and strength.

It is important to develop and/or maintain good muscle strength because it helps ensure good posture (and, in a roundabout way, good digestion and elimination). Good muscle strength makes it easier to carry things from packages to grandkids. And toned muscles can mean less injury.

I mentioned earlier that people lose 20 percent of their muscle tissue by the time they are sixty-five years old. So naturally, with that muscle loss comes loss of muscle strength. Fortunately, muscle strength can be improved by "overloading" the muscle, making it work harder than it is used to working. This can be done by repeating a motion many times or by making the muscle lift more weight than it is used to lifting. Both of these methods can make the muscle sore, so be careful not to overdo it. This is one of the reasons that in a good exercise program, days of rest are scheduled in between days that include workouts.

Balance

As you move through the day, your body is usually off balance. For instance, whenever you take a step you are off balance, but your body has learned to quickly counterbalance so you don't fall. As you get older, your ability to counterbalance slows because messages from the brain to the body are slowed a bit. This delay increases the chance of mishap and injury.

Good balance, important to all of us, is affected by internal as well as external factors. The internal factors have to do with sensory receptors such as vision and hearing. For instance, when eyesight diminishes, depth perception decreases. With side vision impaired, simple tasks such as climbing stairs can be a problem. Quick and sudden head motion can disturb the fluid in the inner ear, causing loss of balance.

To move with agility and safety, you have to be aware of your body. This body awareness, or *kinesthetic sense*, depends on the nervous system and muscles acting as an integrated unit. If you were to walk on a balance beam, you would use your eyes to help you walk a straight line. But if you were to close your eyes, your kinesthetic sense would take over.

Kinesthetic sense can be improved with physical activity. This fact is especially important for those who are coping with poor eyesight and hearing problems.

Agility

A good overall exercise program should improve and maintain agility. Even simple daily activities require that we move easily and quickly. Everyday living requires that all of us be ready for the unexpected: moving out of the way of a child riding a bicycle on the sidewalk, dodging a shopping cart at the supermarket—quick moves like these are all in a day's work. The ability to artfully dodge what is coming at you can lessen your chance of injury (the injury from being hit or from pulling a muscle while trying to get out of the way).

Coordination

Coordination is simply using the right muscles at the right time. As we age, our fine motor coordination isn't always up to par. This can be a nuisance when we attempt such tasks as writing, sewing, or picking up change from a counter. Simple hand exercises can improve the fine motor coordination necessary for these tasks, while rhythmical exercises that work the arms and legs can improve general body coordination.

Range of Motion

The range of motion from full movement in one direction to full movement in the other is often referred to as joint flexibility. For some joints, the bony structure limits the flexibility (elbows, knees, etc.). Sometimes flexibility is limited by the amount of muscle you have. (Some athletes have developed their upper-arm muscles to such an extent that it limits their arm movements.)

In still other joints, such as the ankles, hip, or back, flexibility is limited (or not limited) by the condition of the soft tissues (muscles and connective tissues). Because soft tissue can be modified by physical methods, they are important in the effort to fend off aches and pains.

Reaction Time

Reaction time, the time it takes the brain to send a message to the muscles, slows as we age. Our ability to react quickly affects any situation. When driving a car or even crossing the street, our reaction time is important for our safety. Women volunteers from Leisure World, aged fifty-seven to eighty-five, participated in a general exercise class three times a week for three years to test the effects of exercise on movement, coordination, balance, and reaction time. The results indicated that regular physical exercise improved reaction time and all the other parameters mentioned (Rikli & Edwards, 1991).

The Amazing Hulda Crooks

Hulda Crooks of Loma Linda, California is a 91-year-old who enjoys mountain climbing. Around Mt. Whitney, east of Fresno, Hulda is a local heroine and something of a legend for her hiking accomplishments, which would be impressive at any age. Hulda has conquered the 14,495 foot high Mt. Whitney (the highest mountain in the United States, this side of Alaska) twenty-two times since 1962, and recently she completed a climb of the 12,388 foot high Mount Fuji in Japan (Cooper, 1987).

I know the difficulty that Mount Whitney can present to a hiker because my husband, two daughters, and I have hiked Hulda's route. It's not something you decide to do on a whim because you have nothing to do on a Sunday afternoon. We prepared for a year, walking local trails in heavy protective boots that weighed five pounds each. The trail to the top of Mount Whitney is not a kind one; it is steep in some places and narrow in others. Occasionally, spots can be found that are both. The ten-and-a-half mile trail is littered with broken rocks. Aside from these obstacles, walking with your head in the clouds can also take its toll on your body. As you approach 10,000 feet, the air becomes noticeably thin. As you climb toward the peak, there is less oxygen available for your body and your body reacts. You breathe faster, and, in the higher altitude, you get tired faster.

It took the four of us (my husband, our daughters, and me) two days to climb Mount Whitney. A young, healthy adult could make the climb in a day. A reasonable plan for the climb might be to allow one day at base camp to adjust, one day to make the climb to the top, and one day to return.

A tiny lady with an ever-present smile and snowy hair, Hulda refuses to see fitness and aging as incompatible. "There's nothing special about me. I just work at health instead of whiling away my time sitting in a rocking chair," she says (Cooper, 1987).

DRESSING FOR THE OCCASION

I hope by now that exercise is beginning to sound pretty good to you. But before you go after that accelerated heart rate, there are a few things you should know.

Clothing

What you wear during exercise depends on where and when you exercise. It will change with time, place, and season.

Cold Weather

If you're exercising outside in cold weather, be sure to dress in light layers. You might start with a shirt or blouse, add a light sweater, and top with a coat. The layers will trap the heat next to the skin, and as your body heats up they will be easy to remove.

Wet Weather

When your body gets wet, either from perspiration or rain, you lose the heat built up by the body through exercise. Even if you're wearing layered clothing, wet layers will not do you any good. If you suspect the skies are going to part and give you a good dousing, prepare for it by taking an umbrella or by wearing waterproof (not plastic, which accelerates dehydration) clothing. I think daily exercise is important, and I tell my students who walk for their daily dose of exercise that they should get up and out, *rain or shine*! If the weather is really bad, exercise indoors. Check with your local mall, many of them offer walking programs.

Hot Weather

When you hit your own personal "boiling point" during hot weather, you'll have to decide what clothing—or lack of clothing—feels good to you. Here are a few tips to help you make a personal decision on what to wear.

- Clothing made of rubber or plastic causes moisture to build on the skin. I consider plastic exercise suits dangerous, for they accelerate dehydration of the body. I won't let people wear them in my classes.

- Exercise outfits made of cotton are recommended. Cotton fabric absorbs moisture better than other material. Cotton exercise outfits should be loose-fitting, so the air is free to circulate between your skin and your clothing.

- Light-colored clothing is more desirable because dark colors absorb more heat.

Indoor Exercising

What you wear for indoor exercise classes is a personal decision. Keep in mind that you will undoubtedly work up some body heat as you go through your routine. Naturally, pick an outfit that works for you: shorts and a top, a warm-up suit, or a snazzy leotard with matching tights. Choose something comfortable (there's no advantage to grimacing through you routines). I recommend layering because layered clothing can be removed as your body warms up.

Shoes

The kind of shoes you wear for your exercise routine is very important. In the case of exercise, one shoe cannot fit all needs. Thank goodness shoe manufacturers have recognized this and have come out with shoes specifically designed for different exercise routines.

For walking, you'll need shoes that support a straight-ahead, heel-to-toe motion. It's important for this type of shoe to be cushioned to absorb the stress on ankles, hips, knees, and lower back.

For an aerobics or exercise class, your shoes should provide good support during side-to-side moves. Walking shoes should be cushioned.

Remember, shoes for general use cannot give you the support and cushion needed for today's exercise programs. Select shoes designed to prevent injury. They may cost a little more, but they are worth it.

Socks

I often see sock violations in my classes committed by those who have not yet learned that the right socks are important for good foot health. Nylon hose is a "no-no" because it traps moisture; nylon knee-highs are worse because they trap moisture while the knee band cuts off circulation.

Do buy yourself a few good pairs of exercise socks. They should be both cotton, to absorb perspiration, and cushioned, to buffer the impact of movement on a non-giving surface.

THE ENVIRONMENT

Start walking on level areas. As your fitness improves, you can take on some hills. (You can determine your fitness level by monitoring your heart rate, page 69.) Who knows, you may even end up taking the high road in the mountains like Hulda Crooks (page 29)!

For any outdoor exercise, I tell my students to exercise before 10:00 a.m. or after the sun has gone down. This way the air they breathe won't be as heavily tainted by heat and pollution. I also recommend avoiding heavily trafficked streets because of the auto exhaust fumes.

CHAPTER 4

Designing Your Own Program

The idea that exercise is good for your health is so simple many can't believe the good news. Perhaps my recommendation would be more readily accepted if I came up with a costly pill, an expensive treatment, or some bizarre concept, like the rejuvenating effects of hanging topsy-turvy with bats during an eclipse. But I can't. I can only tell you what other professionals and I have observed. Aerobic exercise lowers blood pressure, reduces the risk of heart attacks and strokes, and improves overall heart and lung function. A good exercise program can tone muscles, enhance motor coordination, and help make you physically fit. A physically fit body has energy, stamina, and strength. Physically fit people are able to do anything they want all day long, with enough get-up-and-go in reserve in case of an emergency.

The idea of becoming physically fit through exercise has obviously been on your mind, or you wouldn't have selected this book. Congratulations on your first commitment to a better you!

SUCCESS—ONE STEP AT A TIME

Set Reasonable Goals

Think of your fitness program as a series of stepping stones that lead to a first goal, then a second, and so on, until you achieve your major goal. Let me clarify this with an example.

Let's say you need to lose thirty pounds. If you constantly think of yourself as someone who's waddling around with thirty pounds of excess baggage, you'll soon convince yourself that your small changes are fruitless and that getting fit is hopeless. Quit looking at the—pardon the expression—big picture. Instead, think of your projected weight loss in reasonable increments, say one pound a week, and set your goal accordingly: "At the end of three weeks, I hope to lose three pounds." With this temporary commitment, three pounds have now become your focus.

If, at the end of three weeks, you've only lost one and one-half pounds, pat yourself on the back for that victory, and re-enlist in a new commitment program. You may have to accelerate your exercise program from three days a week to four, five, or six, but this small step will help ensure success.

The Buddy System

A good friend is indispensable to anyone undertaking an exercise program. An understanding friend can be a coach, a cheerleader, and a co-celebrant during the successes. A friend can listen sympathetically when the pounds are clinging; walk with you through rain, sleet, and snow; and slap your wrist when you are reaching for the donut!

Reap the Rewards

As you achieve each goal, reward yourself. Buy yourself that book you've been wanting to read, have a picnic, go to the beach, buy some new clothes. Anything—except a hot fudge sundae—is fair game. Recognize the fact that you've made some progress and celebrate!

All three: a goal, a friend, and a reward are critical to a successful fitness program. That's why they appear in our fitness contract (pages 36 and 37).

THE PROGRAM FOR YOU

You can figure what areas you need to work on by taking notes on those movements and actions that give you trouble. Are you limber enough to touch you toes? Can you do arm circles without feeling strain? Can you reach behind your back? How many minutes of aerobics can you do without feeling "winded"? You won't have difficulty finding your weak spots. Weak links make themselves known. You're probably already aware of the areas that need attention even without giving yourself the acid test! Once you've pinpointed these areas, you can select from the exercises provided in Part Two of this book to personalize your program.

I recommend an exercise program that includes both aerobic activity and a conditioning exercise program. There are many aerobic activities from which to choose. Walking, jogging, swimming, hiking in the hills, or riding a bicycle are all excellent. In fact, I recently saw a news report on a couple in their seventies who surf! Pick whatever aerobic activity pleases you and be sure to do it at least three days a week. Chapter 5 gives detailed information on aerobic exercise. On the other days, you can work on specific muscles with some specific conditioning exercise routines (see Chapters 6 and 7).

If you're just starting out, ten minutes of exercise is enough. When that becomes comfortable for you, add one minute to your exercise session each time you work out. It won't be long before you're doing thirty, forty, fifty, and even sixty minutes of exercise. And you'll never be your "old self" again.

YOU'VE GOTTEN READY AND SET, NOW IT'S TIME TO GO!

The most important thing to remember is—*if you don't use it you will lose it.* Research has now found that most problems of older age, once attributed to the aging process, are actually due to disease, abuse, and *lack of use.* You alone are responsible for taking charge of your own health, so become informed, aware, and active. Decide on some aerobic fun and go for it. Choose an activity found on the Aerobic Exercise Program (page 72); select some specific conditioning exercises from Chapters 6 and 7. Keep track of your progress on the Personal Fitness Chart on page 39. This record keeping will be an incentive for you to get out and get going!

Putting Your Best Foot Forward

Walking is a great exercise for anyone at any age. If you walk an hour a day at a brisk pace, you should, during this physical activity, burn the 2,000-weekly calories that should be expended through physical activity

Sample Contract

I, *Hilda Healthy*, am committed to beginning a fitness program. I will *walk 10 minutes daily* the first week. During the second week I will *swim every other day*. In addition, I have agreed to the following things:

I will walk in the morning.
I will exercise 3 times a week.
I will record my progress daily.

When my warm-up, exercise, and cool down reach a total of thirty minutes, I will reward myself *with a new outfit.*

*   *   *

I, *Fanny Friend*, agree to be *Hilda*'s friend, helper, cheerleader, and coach as he/she undertakes a new exercise program. As a wearer of these many hats, I promise to:

1. *Accompany Hilda on walks.*
2. *Support Hilda's efforts to become fit.*
3. *Help Hilda set new goals in 3 weeks.*

Signed: *Hilda Healthy*   Date: *9-7-92*
Helper: *Fanny Friend*   Renewal Date: *9-28-92*

My Contract

I, _____, am committed to beginning a fitness
program. I will _____ the first week.
During the second week I will_____.
In addition, I have agreed to the following things:

_____

_____

_____

When my warm-up, exercise, and cool down reach a total of
thirty minutes, I will reward myself _____

_____

*   *   *

I, _____ , agree to be _____'s
friend, helper, cheerleader, and coach as he/she undertakes a
new exercise program. As a wearer of these many hats,
I promise to:

    1._____

    2._____

    3._____

Signed:_____ Date: _____

Helper: _____ Renewal Date: _____

to keep your heart in good shape. Research done at Stanford University indicates that daily aerobic exercise is a much-preferred antidote to heart disease than the exercise spurts usually reserved for weekends (Wood, 1986).

Walking can be your aerobic workout. Don't start off in high gear, rather increase your effort at certain intervals (see page 72). Some people can walk around the house or complete daily chores without having any leg problems, but during a brisk walk or a bicycle ride, they might experience leg pain. Not enough oxygen reaches their legs during the extra-effort activity.

I encourage my students to walk through leg pain with a deliberate heel-to-toe foot motion. Although the pain will still visit from time to time, exercise can improve this tendency. Some of my students, by increasing their exercise slowly, have gotten their walking up to four and five miles without experiencing leg trouble.

On Walking

HELPFUL HINTS

- *Start with a flat course.*
- *Vary your routes.*
- *Do not stride too fast. You should be able to carry on a conversation while you walk. Do not become breathless.*
- *Be consistent. Make walking a positive addiction.*
- *Wear good shoes with proper cushioning.*
- *Wait at least an hour after meals before walking.*
- *Wear loose-fitting clothes.*

TO AVOID INJURY

- *If your arthritis flares up, walk at a slower pace.*
- *If you get pain in your lower leg, walk "heel-to-toe, heel-to-toe" at a slower rate.*
- *If you get pains in the front of your lower leg, check your shoes to make sure they have good cushioning.*
- *If you develop dizziness, chest pain, cold sweats, or nausea, **see your physician immediately!***

KEEPING TRACK
PERSONAL FITNESS CHART

1. Enter the activity and date performed under the appropriate columns.
2. During the activity period, take your pulse (page 70) and establish your Exercising Heart Rate.
3. During the cool-down period, establish your Ending Heart Rate and record it.
4. Under the Time column, record the number of minutes exercised in your Training Zone (page 67).
5. Evaluate how you felt when exercising (eg. tired, weak, invigorated, energetic, etc.) and enter under the Effort column.

Date	Activity	Exercising Heart Rate	Ending Heart Rate	Time	Effort

Susan: Exercise and Blood Pressure

When Susan came to see me at the fitness center at Leisure World, she was quite distressed. Her doctor had just taken her blood pressure, and the reading was unacceptably high. She had to do something to get the pressure down or she would have to go on medication. Susan had exercised regularly in the past, but since the death on her husband, six months earlier, she had stopped going to class.

What Susan needed was some aerobic exercise. She decided that walking would be her exercise of choice. I suggested she begin her walking program in the fitness center so we could easily monitor her. She began walking on a treadmill three days a week. After she was able to walk effortlessly for thirty minutes without stopping, Susan began walking in her neighborhood. I also suggested she begin doing some relaxation exercises to reduce the level of her emotional stress.

While Susan worked on lowering her blood pressure, we monitored her carefully. Within six weeks, we began to notice a positive change. Not only had she lost ten pounds, her blood pressure had dropped and her self-esteem had improved.

When it was time to see her doctor, Susan was anxious. She soon learned, however, that her exercising had paid off. Susan's doctor was happy to inform her that her blood pressure was in an acceptable range, and she would not have to go on any medication. The doctor told a relieved Susan, "Just keep doing what you're doing."

Heart Smart

The average heart beats 40 million times a year. Each day, with about 100,000 contractions, an average of 2,500 gallons of blood is pumped through this incredible powerhouse. In its operation, the heart services many thousands of miles of blood vessels in the average adult. One researcher calculated that the heart muscles work twice as hard as the leg muscles of a person who is running. While we can always sit down and rest when most of our body muscles are tired, we cannot rest the heart. The heart keeps going as long as we live. A phenomenally efficient and durable muscle, the heart gets only a fraction of a second of rest between beats.

It is important to recognize that the heart is indeed a muscle. So, as a leg muscle might be strengthened and improved by exercise, so might the heart muscle. Over the past several decades, research has indicated that exercise enhances heart functioning.

Exercise and Heart Attacks

Those who have suffered from coronary disease or heart attacks can benefit impressively with specially designed exercise programs. Dr. Gottheiner in Israel, Dr. Hellerstein in Cleveland, Drs. Kasch and Boyer in San Diego, and other experts have developed exercise programs designed to assist the recuperating heart patient. Their results have been nothing short of outstanding. Men who previously would have been encouraged to become "cardiac invalids," have been able to return to pre-heart-attack levels of activity. Many developed far more vigor than they had before their illness.

If you have a history of heart trouble, it is imperative that you first check with your doctor before beginning an exercise program. Once you have your doctor's approval, choose a program that best suits you.

Breathing Easier

With age, the flexibility of the rib cage, especially in women, decreases. It can become more difficult to take deep breaths and to fill the lungs to capacity. The rib cage just doesn't give as easily. If you took a balloon, placed it in a glass bottle, then tried to inflate it, you might better understand what happens to the lungs when the rib cage is not flexible.

Many people with breathing difficulties due to a less flexible rib cage or from complications such as asthma, emphysema, and allergies are naturally reluctant to exercise because it is hard for them to breathe during any kind of accelerated physical activity. The already small airways to the lungs are blocked, making it difficult to move air in and out. Many people with lung complications "play it safe" and sit on the sidelines of any physical activity; but the truth is, it would be better for those with lung problems to get out of the bleachers and into the action. People with lung problems need to keep exercising to prevent further loss of breathing capacity. Most important, the proper exercise can actually bolster impaired lung capacity. Chronic wheezing, coughing, and breathlessness can take the fun out of life and whittle away at self-confidence.

Anyone with breathing problems should become involved in some form of aerobic exercising. Concentration on exercises that increase the flexibility of the rib cage, strengthen the abdominal muscles, and tune-up the muscles along the sides of the body are most beneficial. Strong muscles encourage good posture, and give the lungs breathing room. Table 4.1 offers an effective program to increase one's breathing capacity.

Blood Pressure

Blood pressure has been called the "barometer" of good health. It can help forecast a person's health much like actual barometers aid in forecasting the weather. National statistics show clear-cut relationships between high blood pressure (hypertension) and disease.

Have you ever asked yourself why your doctor is so concerned about your blood pressure? For starters, the relationship between blood pressure and the heart is similar to that of air pressure in a tire. If the pressure is too high, the danger of a blowout is greater. A human "blowout" would be a stroke or an aneurysm, but there are other, equally important high blood pressure effects you should know about.

Hank: Breathing Easier

Hank, at age fifty-two, was the youngest participant in Dr. deVries' initial research at Leisure World. While Hank's breathing capacity only improved by a mere 15 percent, his gain was extremely important. Hank started the program with a breathing capacity comparable to a sixty-three-year-old. After forty-two weeks of the exercise program, his breathing capacity was in the forty-five-year-old range (deVries, 1974).

Hank's good results are important for anyone who struggles with breathing problems. It's never too late to be better than you are!

Table 4.1   Program to Enhance Breathing Capacity

Exercise	Beginning	Intermediate	Advanced
Overhead Arm and Torso Stretch	Hold 10 seconds	Hold 20 seconds	Hold 30 seconds
Upper-Back and Chest Stretch	3 repetitions	5 repetitions	10 repetitions
Side Stretch	Hold 10 seconds	Hold 20 seconds	Hold 30 seconds
Rib Stretch	3 repetitions	5 repetitions	10 repetitions
Trunk Twister	Hold 10 seconds	Hold 20 seconds	Hold 30 seconds
Abdominal Pushes	3 repetitions	5 repetitions	10 repetitions
Abdominal Hand Pushes	3 repetitions	5 repetitions	10 repetitions
Leg Lifts	3 repetitions	5 repetitions	10 repetitions

The heart functions similarly to an ordinary pump that might pump water. As the heart tries to maintain the flow of blood and oxygen to the body, different situations bring about different demands. Sometimes this pump might be required to provide a greater flow rate; other times, it might be necessary to increase pressure. If something on the inside of the artery resists smooth flow, then the heart must exert greater pressure. Many experiments concerning flow rate and pressure have been done with the heart. Results show that the heart is not strained at all by the demand for increased flow rates alone, but strain on the heart increases when the blood pressure is increased. If blood pressure is chronically too high, the added strain on the heart is constant.

Increased blood pressure can also create problems by damaging the interior blood vessel walls, making them more likely to become clogged. Plaque can build on artery walls. This build-up, or a piece of it, can break off and clog an artery. If this clogging occurs in a blood vessel that supplies the heart with blood, a heart attack can occur; if it occurs in a blood vessel in the brain, the result is a stroke (Morehouse et al, 1971).

Rules for Those with High Blood Pressure

- Exercise, walk, or ride a stationary bike at your own speed (see page 72). Your breathing will be your best guide. You should be able to talk to someone while exercising.
- Never exercise if you are feeling breathless.
- Stay at any one level of exercise until you are comfortable moving up. Move ahead only if you feel ready.
- Allow for a day of rest between exercise days. Exercising on Monday, Wednesday, and Friday, or on Tuesday, Thursday, and Saturday will provide the needed day of rest.
- If your systolic pressure (top number) is higher than 200 or your diastolic pressure (lower number) is over 95, you should not exercise without checking with your doctor.

Stress

When we are under stress, our bodies produce stress hormones. These hormones cause our blood pressure to rise, our heartbeat to increase, and our body to tense for action. This reaction, which is also referred to as our *fight or flight response*, was applicable in the Stone Age when stress was more easily defined. In those days, a wild boar might attack and man would have to make the decision to fight or run, but the confrontation would be resolved and the body could get back to normal. Not so today.

While it is unliklely that we will face a wild boar on our patio, it *is* likely that we might sit in traffic during rush hour. As we sit, we might become late for an important appointment or a plane flight—and all we can do is fume! If we're not stuck on the freeway, we might be jousting with a computer over bills or a bank account. Frankly, it might be easier to take on the wild boar!

Tension Can Make You Physically Sick

What exactly is this spoiler called nervous tension? In general, it's the result of combatting our environment. Our surroundings have evolved from the peacefulness of an agricultural atmosphere to the highly complex, fast-paced, crowded, and intense hustle-bustle that comes with industry.

A certain amount of tension is necessary. We all have deadlines, and because of pressure things get done. Not stress, but *distress* can create problems. Some tension is necessary to life; too much tension is destructive.

You have only to look around to see immediately how our senses can become overtaxed and battered by our surroundings. City noise from traffic, aircrafts, radios, and televisions constantly pummels our ears. Smog assaults our eyes and noses. Urban overcrowding concentrates, accentuates, and augments these harrassments of our senses. In addition to this, we can have personal problems. Sickness, divorce, loneliness, and the loss of friends and relatives can all add to the pressures in our lives.

With progress comes change, and time and again we have found ourselves victims of these changes and "pressured" into adapting. Money machines at banks, computerized libraries, and self-service gas pumps are just a few minor examples of how modern changes add pressure to our lives. A daily source of sensory overstimulation can be found on our crowded roads and freeways. Freeway driving requires constant sensory feedback, rapid-fire decisions, and, oftentimes, lightning-quick moves. It can be nerve-wracking.

In order to understand how the mental and physical barrage on our nervous system affects us, let's consider a simple reflex called the *startle reflex*. If someone shoots off a firecracker in a crowd, the individual response can vary from mild annoyance to near hysteria. Further, the effect on any one individual will vary from day to day. For example, on the day when a person has worked under relatively serene conditions, he might barely react to the firecracker. However, if that same person has been working under the additional strain of a jackhammer's noise all day, the same firecracker explosion might cause a wild jump or even tears.

The bad news is that a constantly stressed condition takes its toll. Health problems such as heart attacks, high blood pressure, ulcers, high cholesterol, back problems, headaches, and immune-deficiency diseases, result from a constantly stressed condition. The good news is that researchers report that improved physical fitness is accompanied by a significant drop in blood pressure and improved health (Selve, 1956).

Anyone suffering from stress should first be examined by his physician. Once any physical causes are ruled out, a fitness program can be started. An aerobics program that includes walking, biking, or swimming will di-

Stress: Carl's Story

Carl, at sixty-eight years old, was a jewelry manufacturer. The tension-creating task of operating his business in the face of stiff competition, coupled with virtually no physical activity during most of his life, took a toll on Carl's health and well-being as he approached retirement age. For years, he had suffered from very severe tension headaches, averaging three or four headaches a week. He admits he "ate aspirins like peanuts" for relief.

When Carl started the deVries exercise program (Chapter 1), his tests showed that the electrical activity in his muscles was higher than average. In short, Carl was a tense person. After five months of physical conditioning, his muscular electrical activity decreased to 37 percent of what it had been, and he no longer suffered from headaches. But this is not where Carl's story ends.

Feeling much better than he had in a long time, Carl went on a motoring vacation. After ten days of traveling (and no exercise) Carl's severe headaches returned. He began exercising again (as best he could) while on the road. Again his headaches disappeared (deVries, 1974).

It would be hard to claim exercise as the cure for all headaches, but this is what happened to one man, and it has also happened to others. On the average, the participants in the program reduced their resting muscle activity by about 10 percent.

minish body tension. The movements performed in an exercise conditioning program are also helpful. Start with the Sit-Down Workout (Chapter 6). When you are comfortable doing these exercises, progress to the more difficult exercises in the General Conditioning Workout (Chapter 7).

Conquering Fatigue

"I tire easily. . . . " "I'm always dragging. . . ." "I don't seem to have any energy. . . ." Physicians will tell you that these are common complaints heard frequently from older patients. More often than not, regardless of the primary reason for the office visit, older patients complain of persistent fatigue.

I always ask my exercisers what they feel the most important result of the conditioning program is for them. The most commonly heard answer is, "more energy, less fatigue."

How do we account for this relief from fatigue and tiredness brought about by a better level of physical fitness? Several factors contribute to the renewed energy enjoyed by the participants, but increased physical activity heads the list.

As you might remember, improved fitness through exercise makes the complex process of transporting oxygen throughout the human system more efficient. With good physical fitness, greater qualities of oxygen are available to the muscles. A person's energy level depends on the availability of oxygen to the active tissues. This is because vigorous physical activity can be sustained only a minute or two without oxygen. Oxygen is a necessary factor for the burning of foodstuffs stored in the muscles. Any prolonged action of a muscle in the body depends on this process, called *oxidation,* to generate a unit of energy. Any move you make, whether it is wiggling your index finger, using your large leg muscles when running, or using your long arm muscles when playing tennis, depends on the availability of oxygen in the muscles. You must burn foodstuffs that are stored in the muscles or supplied by the blood to produce energy. And you must have oxygen "on the spot" to burn the foodstuffs.

A person who has not engaged in much hard physical activity during the course of the day might question how the emphasis on greater muscle demand could be the answer to fatigue. Unless you're flat on your back, your muscles are working all day long. If you are a tense person, your muscles might even be working to some degree when you're lying down. Muscle fatigue can manifest itself as tightness in the lower back, even if a person is doing nothing more strenuous than standing still. The fact is that even the slightest effort can quickly produce muscle fatigue in poorly conditioned muscles.

Fortunately, muscle function can be improved by appropriate exercises. Studies indicate that persons with less strength initially, show the greatest improvement after exercising.

First, check with your doctor to rule out any medical problems that might cause fatigue. If your doctor cannot find a physical reason for your tired feeling, why not work on conditioning your muscles so they don't give up so easily? A walking or biking program would be a great start. The Aerobic Exercise Program (page 72) is great for jump-starting tired bodies.

This can be combined with the Sit-Down Workout (Chapter 6) or the General Conditioning Workout (Chapter 7).

Joint Stiffness

Use it or lose it. That pretty much sums up my advice on keeping your body well. Joint stiffness, due to lack of use, hinders posture and movement much like an old gate that is difficult to open and close because of a rusty hinge. Because of time and disuse, the hinge has become balky and stiff. Our bodies can become like that gate.

If we don't move our joints through all possible ranges of motion, we will lose some of our potential for movement. Then we will find ourselves caught in a vicious cycle: lack of movement causes the joint to lose its range of motion; the loss causes pain when an attempt is made to move the joint; and pain discourages any effort to move. It is an established fact that when a muscle is not worked through a normal range of movement on a regular basis, the connective tissue around the joint becomes short and can become injured more easily.

Recently, a series of experiments at Johns Hopkins Medical School resulted in the following conclusion:

Joint stiffness resides primarily in the muscles and connective tissues that serve to move the joints, rather than in the joint structure itself.

Table 4.2 provides a Joint Flexibility Program. Diligently following the suggested exercises will help your joints maintain maximum range of motion.

Lower-Back Pain

Connective tissue does what it sounds like it does—it holds the body together. Connective tissue binds muscles to bones with tendons, and bone to bone with ligaments; it covers and unites muscles with a sheet of fibrous tissue beneath the surface of the skin. In general, connective tissue forms a framework for all the organs and for the body as a whole. These tendons, ligaments, and fibrous tissues extend less with age, giving the impression of stiffness. Research shows that for every decade after the age of forty, we lose about 4 percent of our flexibility, but this same decrease in flexibility can also be brought about as the result of immobilization.

Table 4.2   Joint Flexibility Program

Exercise	Beginning	Intermediate	Advanced
Shoulder Stretch 2	Hold 15 seconds	Hold 30 Seconds	Hold 30 seconds
Leg Stretch	Hold 15 seconds	Hold 30 seconds	Hold 30 seconds
Overhead Arm Stretch	Hold 15 seconds	Hold 30 seconds	Hold 30 seconds
Lower-Back Stretch	Hold 15 seconds	Hold 30 seconds	Hold 30 seconds
Hip Stretch	Hold 15 seconds	Hold 30 seconds	Hold 30 seconds
Straight-Leg Stretch	Hold 15 seconds	Hold 30 seconds	Hold 30 seconds
Side-Straddle Stretch	Hold 15 seconds	Hold 30 seconds	Hold 30 seconds
Soles-Together Stretch	Hold 15 seconds	Hold 30 seconds	Hold 30 seconds
Trunk Twister	Hold 15 seconds	Hold 30 seconds	Hold 30 seconds
Rib and Waist Stretch	Hold 10 seconds	Hold 20 seconds	Hold 30 seconds
Torso Twister	Hold 10 seconds	Hold 20 seconds	Hold 30 seconds
Side Stretch	3 repetitions	5 repetitions	10 repetitions

When the sheet of fibrous tissue shortens due to age or lack of exercise, it places undue pressure on nerve pathways, causing aches and pains. With muscle pain, a *splinting reflex* (an effort to immobilize the muscle by making it contract) occurs. Unfortunately, this contraction shortens the muscle again and the whole area can go into muscle spasm. Low-back pain typifies the "pain-contraction-shortened muscle-pain" cycle.

Many people suffer with back pain. If you're one of them, *never start an exercise program without first conferring with your doctor.* Once you get your physician's approval, refer to Table 4.3 and follow these four tips:

• Perform all recommended exercises slowly and with deliberate motions.
• Take a deep breath before and after each exercise set.

- Do only three repetitions of each exercise.
- Perform your program once a day, *every day.*

The Senior Image

Some of the worst stereotyping of seniors involves their physical image. Remember Arte Johnson's old-man character on the television show *Laugh-In*? He was everything any of us would hate to be—a sniveling, drooling,

Table 4.3   Back Exercise Program

Exercise	Beginning	Intermediate	Advanced
Exercises for the Neck (all but Looking-Up)	3 repetitions	5 repetitions	10 repetitions
Shoulder Shrugs	3 repetitions	5 repetitions	10 repetitions
Upper-Back and Chest Stretch	3 repetitions	5 repetitions	10 repetitions
Abdominal Pushes	3 repetitions	5 repetitions	10 repetitions
Leg Lowering*	3 repetitions	5 repetitions	10 repetitions
Sit-Ups*	3 repetitions	5 repetitions	10 repetitions
	Do not attempt to sit all the way up! Lying flat, curl your upper body forward and up. Keep your chin on your chest. Roll forward until you feel your abdomen tighten like it is squeezing water from a sponge.		
Knee-to-Chest Stretch	3 repetitions	5 repetitions	10 repetitions
Lower-Back Stretch	Hold 10 seconds	Hold 20 seconds	Hold 30 seconds
Straight-Leg Stretch	Hold 10 seconds	Hold 20 seconds	Hold 30 seconds
Soles-Together Stretch	Hold 10 seconds	Hold 20 seconds	Hold 30 seconds

*More advanced versions of Sit-Ups and Leg Lowering can be tried in six to eight weeks.

letching, forgetful old idiot. And he shuffled around, back bent and eyes riveted to the ground with the flexibility of a robot.

Johnson played the stereotype beautifully. I know where he got his material for the character because, unfortunately, I have seen what aging can do to people. I've seen the withered frames and the bent backs, but I'm happy to report that these common changes in posture and gait do not necessarily have to accompany the aging process (provided the person does not suffer from a significant disease of the joints). I can show you many women and men in their seventies and eighties who, thanks to an individualized physical-fitness routine, stand and walk erect and have a youthful spring in their stride. Even better, I can point out 80-plus-year-olds who run and swim as well.

Weight Control

Americans, more than any others, wage a continual "battle of the bulge." And they do it in some pretty peculiar—and dangerous—ways.

I've seen plastic suits guaranteed to take off those unwanted pounds, creams that promise to melt away body fat, night pills that supposedly help you lose weight as you sleep, and bath potions guaranteed to make you skinny while you're in the tub. The back pages of romance magazines and the Sunday newspaper supplements are jam packed with promises of instant, new, slimmer physiques. Mail-order tablets promise to "shrink your fat cells," "transform you from fat to thin in record time," or "help you lose eight to twenty-five pounds in a week." Losing weight quickly,

---

Irene and the Aquadettes

Irene learned to swim when she was seventy-five years old. She became so good in the water that she joined the Aquadettes, a group of women in their sixties, seventies, and eighties who put on a synchronized swimming show. These ladies practice three times a week; when it gets close to show time they practice every night. They've performed at Lawrence Welk's hotel in Escondido, California and have also been featured on the cover of the National Enquirer.

Matthew and Weight Loss

Sixty-seven-year-old Matthew, who was considerably overweight, began an exercise program at Leisure World. Matthew combined his exercise program with a calorie-restricted diet. Six months into the program he had lost twenty-five pounds.

In his earlier attempt to lose weight, Matthew had undertaken a rigorous diet without exercise. Even though Matthew's unwanted weight had dropped during this first attempt, Matthew felt chronically tired and had little or no energy to do much of anything. Out-of-state friends, whom he saw only periodically, commented on his poor appearance.

Years later, after his successful diet-and-exercise program at Leisure World, Matthew felt great and had the energy to do things. The same friends, on a subsequent visit, commented on his improved appearance and obvious good health.

one pitch goes on, is simpler than you ever dreamed, especially if you take the "most powerful appetite suppressant available without a prescription." In reality, the only thing that is guaranteed to get thinner is your pocketbook.

These claims sound much too good to be true, and I can't help but raise a few questions. Will I be losing water, muscle, or fat? Will I maintain my new weight, or will the pounds ease back on the minute I'm off the pills or fad diet? Are there side effects, such as nervousness or even high blood pressure? Can I stay on this weight-control approach the rest of my life?

I personally recommend taking off weight the old-fashioned way: working at it with diet and exercise. My experience has been that exercise plays a significant role in reducing and maintaining proper body weight in persons of any age. This has been proven scientifically in many studies over the years.

It's not really weight loss we are after, it's *fat* loss. The two are not the same because of the human body's composition. The body is made of active tissues and inactive tissues. The active tissues include muscles, bones, glands, and internal organs; they actually burn away what we eat. Fat acts as a blanket to protect and insulate the body. We don't want to reduce our active tissues, rather the layer of fat that covers it. Exercise is not a panacea for all obese people. Those with serious weight problems should seek the advice of their doctors for the weight-loss approach that is best for them. *For certain people, medical supervision is an absolute necessity. I recommend a doctor's approval for anyone beginning a weight-loss and exercise program. It is also important that you work with a qualified nutritional expert.*

If your weight has remained pretty stable through the years, you're probably not feeling too anxious about this discussion. It's harder to stay in better shape as you age, so I think it's great when the scale is still your friend, but you might need a little more tuning up than you think. Things might not be just what they seem.

If, at age sixty or seventy, you're maintaining the same weight you did at age twenty, you are now between 12 and 15 percent *overfat*. This is because we lose approximately 3 percent of active tissue per decade. The lost tissue gets replaced by fat. So you might not be overweight, but you could be overfat. Excess fat can lead to problems such as diabetes, high blood pressure, coronary heart disease, gout, and cancer; it can also cause gall bladder, back, and joint-related problems.

If you've decided that you'd like to drop a few pounds, add some exercise to your life. Exercise doubles you pleasure, doubles your fun, and accelerates weight loss. This is because an exercised and trained muscle provides more enzymes, which can quickly and efficiently metabolize fat into energy.

Monitoring every calorie requires the control and dedication of a saint. The truth is, a lot of us love to nibble. And when we're nibbling, we're

Law of the Heavy Cookies

Let's say you decide to have two chocolate cookies, just because they are there! Small inexpensive ones (not the kind mother used to make) would be about 100 calories. If you ate two of these little cookies daily, and those 100 calories were over the caloric intake your body needed, your body's shape would begin to pay the price. In thirty-five days—a little over a month—you would have taken in 3,500 extra calories. In body weight, that equals one pound. In a year, this habit would add ten pounds to your torso.

not paying attention to what we're putting in our mouths. Cookies, chips, and cheese chunks (hmmm, makes you want to get some right now, doesn't it?) are favorite nibbling choices, but all are loaded with calories.

Weight-Loss Tips

All of us, at one time or another, have tried to lose weight, and many of us have gotten discouraged before our weight-loss program had even gotten off the ground. To get rid of fat, certain criteria must be met.

- For sensible weight loss, good nutrition is a must. The American Heart Association and the Diabetes Association offer excellent, healthy food plans for all ages.
- Only aerobic exercise will burn fat.
- Do aerobic exercise at least four times a week. (If you want to improve the function of your heart, lungs, and vascular system, only three days are necessary.) If your excess weight seems determined to stay, increase your aerobic exercise to five or even six times a week.
- To effectively burn fat, your aerobic workout should continue, non-stop, for forty-five minutes. Two twenty-five minute sessions won't do it! Follow the prescribed schedule provided on page 72 to gradually and safely increase your workout time.

Walking and Weight Loss

Many people have been discouraged from using exercise to reduce weight because of misleading "salesmanship." For example, it takes ten hours of walking, (or other ridiculously heavy workloads) to lose one pound. It is indeed undesirable, as well as impossible, to try to lose one pound per day in this fashion. But by stating that walking an extra half hour per day can result in a weight loss of nine pounds per year is more encouraging and makes more sense. It is the "long haul" that counts.

Exercising with an Arthritic Condition

Arthritis affects the joints and the connective tissue. Arthritis hampers movement, so many people with this condition think that an exercise class is the last place on Earth they should be. This is not necessarily true.

The most common forms of arthritis among older adults are the rheumatoid and osteoarthritis types. Pain and swelling often accompany rheumatoid arthritis, so the amount of exercise a person with rheumatoid arthritis can do is often dictated by the severity of the disease. Anyone with arthritis should let comfort be their guide when it comes to exercising.

With arthritis, pain is a constant factor whether you exercise or not, but with exercise comes an increase in joint flexibility. The ability for movement becomes greater, resulting in pain reduction.

If you have arthritis in your hands, try the hand and wrist exercises found in Chapter 6 or 7. If you're intent on weight loss, then your program must include some aerobic exercise at least four days a week. Losing weight often takes pressure off painful back, hips, and knee joints.

Table 4.4   Program for Arthritis Sufferers

Exercise	Beginning	Intermediate	Advanced
Exercises for the Neck (all but Looking-Up)	3 repetitions	5 repetitions	10 repetitions
Shoulder Shrugs	3 repetitions	5 repetitions	10 repetitions
Shoulder Stretch	Hold 10 seconds	Hold 20 seconds	Hold 30 seconds
Exercises for the Hands and Wrists	3 repetitions	5 repetitions	10 repetitions
Abdominal Pushes	3 repetitions	5 repetitions	10 repetitions
Abdominal Hand Pushes	3 repetitions	5 repetitions	10 repetitions
Hip Stretch	Hold 10 seconds	Hold 20 seconds	Hold 30 seconds
Knee-to-Chest Stretch	3 repetitions	5 repetitions	10 repetitions
Lower-Back Stretch	3 repetitions	5 repetitions	10 repetitions
Straight-Leg Stretch	3 repetitions	5 repetitions	10 repetitions
Leg Stretch	3 repetitions	5 repetitions	10 repetitions
Exercises for the Feet and Ankles	3 repetitions	5 repetitions	10 repetitions

Table 4.4 provides a recommended stretching program for arthritis sufferers. When you are ready, refer to Table 5.2, found on page 72, and add an endurance segment to your workout program.

If you suffer from arthritis and want to incorporate exercise into your life, the following suggestions should be considered:

- Rheumatoid arthritics *should not* exercise if joints are aggravated by pain and swelling.
- For osteoarthritics, pain generally exists, whether or not there is movement. Incorporate a lot of stretching motions into routines and exercise at a slow pace.
- Do any or all of the exercises in the Sit-Down Workout (Chapter 6).
- Start slowly and gradually increase the number of repetitions.
- If your joints hurt while you are exercising, try slowing down the pace. With exercise the pain might go away.
- Stop exercising if you feel *excessive* pain, or if the pain from exercising lasts more than twenty-four hours.
- Remember, pain is not gain!

Exercise and Osteoporosis

As a person ages, bones become thin. This thinning process affects more women than men. One out of every five post-menopausal women will experience a gradual loss of bone caused by lack of calcium. This calcium loss is also linked to the collapse of the spine commonly known as *dowager's hump.* The wrists and the hips are also affected by bone loss. Complications from hip fractures, such as blood clots and pneumonia, make hip fractures the twelfth leading cause of death in older women today.

Not all exercise is appropriate for people with osteoporosis because the spinal vertebrae are fragile. This condition definitely affects daily living and recreational choices. Those with osteoporosis should focus on exercises that work the connective tissue, manipulating the tissue so that it pulls and tugs on the arms, hips, and backbones. Research indicates that this type of pulling movement actually increases bone density.

Table 4.5 provides a recommended exercise program for osteoporosis suffers. While exercising, if you feel discomfort, slow down the pace; stop if you need to. Remember, however, to *check with your doctor before beginning any exercise program.*

Table 4.5   **Program for Osteoporosis Sufferers**

Exercise	Beginning	Intermediate	Advanced
Neck Exercises (all but Looking-Up)	3 repetitions	5 repetitions	10 repetitions
Random Arm Movements	3 repetitions	5 repetitions	10 repetitions
Shoulder Stretch	Hold 10 seconds	Hold 20 seconds	Hold 30 seconds
Chair Jogging	3 repetitions	5 repetitions	10 repetitions
Abdominal Pushes	3 repetitions	5 repetitions	10 repetitions
Abdominal Hand Pushes	3 repetitions	5 repetitions	10 repetitions
Hip Stretch	Hold 10 seconds	Hold 20 seconds	Hold 30 seconds
Knee-to-Chest Stretch	3 repetitions	5 repetitions	10 repetitions
Straight-Leg Hold	Hold 10 seconds	Hold 20 seconds	Hold 30 seconds
Bent-Arm Raises	3 repetitions	5 repetitions	10 repetitions
Side-Leg Raises	3 repetitions	5 repetitions	10 repetitions

Exercise and Diabetes

Many people can lower their blood sugar level and control their diabetes through exercise and diet. Diabetics can and should exercise, but their diets, food intake, and exercise programs must be balanced to avoid low blood sugar, which could lead to insulin shock.

An active aerobics program (as suggested on page 72) is important for the diabetic because it enhances circulation and gives the heart and arteries a good workout. All exercises found in the Sit-Down and the General Conditioning Workouts (Chapters 6 and 7) are excellent for the diabetic, but special attention should be given to exercises for the legs and the feet.

Any diabetic, but especially diabetics who use insulin injections to control their diabetes, *should consult their doctor before beginning an exercise program.*

A FINAL WORD

Through the years, I have seen just about every type of physical problem. I am convinced that everyone can exercise if he wants to. Begin with a handful of exercises and add more when you feel up to it. Before you know it you will be feeling better and have more energy and less pain. Now that you have been given the tools to design your own personal exercise program, it's time for the exercises.

PART TWO

Your Gateway to Independence

Overview

Now it's time for you to get down to business! Part Two, with its many exercises, supports you through your gateway to independence. Divided into four chapters, Part Two offers the following: "Aerobic Exercise," the "Sit-Down Workout," a "General Conditioning Workout," and "Stretching Exercises."

Chapter 5 offers important guidelines for ensuring an effective aerobic workout. All areas of aerobics are discussed. Information is provided on how to establish heart-rate training zones as well as the importance of a proper warm-up and cool-down period, which are part of a beneficial aerobic workout. Chapter 6 presents the Sit-Down Workout. This program includes exercises that are done while sitting in a chair. It provides a gentle yet effective approach to conditioning. The General Conditioning Workout, found in Chapter 7, is recommended for those in general good health. Designed to condition every part of the body, this workout uses a more strenuous approach than the one found in the Sit-Down Workout. Finally, the Stretching Exercises are presented in Chapter 8. These stretches concentrate on maintaining flexibility of the connective tissue surrounding the joints; they can be done alone or in conjunction with the Aerobic, Sit-Down, or General Conditioning programs.

Whether the program you have selected is the Sit-Down or the General Conditioning Workout, perform the exercises in the order that they are listed. This will ensure a proper warm up as you move along. You may notice that some exercises are repeated in both programs. This is because the exercises will get the job done regardless of whether the modified or the more strenuous approach is being followed. It is very important, however, to select your exercises wisely. Consider your body's strengths and weaknesses when establishing your individual goals and remember: *always check with your doctor or health-care provider before beginning any exercise program.*

As you've been thinking about yourself and imagining the new you, I'm sure you're anxious to get started. I encourage your enthusiasm, but I also don't want your program to be over in a week because exercising turned out to be too much of a chore for you. The following suggestions will help you get right to your problem areas while keeping the fun in your effort to keep fit.

GUIDELINES FOR AN AEROBIC-EXERCISE PROGRAM

- When choosing an aerobic exercise, make sure you select an activity you enjoy (e.g. swimming, biking, walking).
- Your clothing should be comfortable. As you exercise you will probably feel warmer. Wear a jacket or sweater that you can take off should this occur.
- Wear shoes with proper cushioning to prevent any injury to the back, hips, knees, and feet.
- Cotton socks absorb moisture and provide additional cushioning for greater comfort.
- When exercising, always begin your activity slowly, gradually increasing the intensity of your workout.
- Aerobic exercise will increase your heart rate. Your heart rate should not exceed the guidelines given in Chapter 5.
- Aerobic exercise should be done at least three times a week on a regular basis.
- If you want to lose weight, you need to exercise aerobically for a minimum of forty-five minutes, four times a week.
- A day of rest between sessions is recommended when doing aerobic exercise.

GUIDELINES FOR THE SIT-DOWN AND
GENERAL CONDITIONING PROGRAMS

- Allow adequate rest time between individual exercises and between exercise sessions. Tired, sore muscles won't respond if you ask them to work again before they are ready. It is better to underdo than overdo. You don't want soreness or muscle and joint damage. It is far better to finish an exercise session wanting to continue it again, rather than feeling so uncomfortable that you don't ever want to move again.

- Exercising three times a week with a day's rest in between is sufficient to improve strength, flexibility, balance, coordination, agility, and re-action time.

- You do not have to do all the recommended repetitions that are suggested in the Sit-Down and General Conditioning programs. Begin by doing one or two repetitions, and gradually add more until you reach the recommended number.

- It is important to maintain regularity in your exercise program. Skipping sessions can cause injury when you begin again. (If you have skipped sessions, remember to start again slowly.)

- If you feel pain, stop doing that motion. If the pain goes away, slowly try the exercise again. If the pain persists, eliminate that motion and try again later.

The "No Pain, No Gain" Theory

I don't believe in the saying, "No, pain, no gain." In fact, I believe this attitude is downright dangerous. Exercise doesn't have to hurt, nor does it have to be a miserable part of your day, an agonizing "must do." Pick an activity or activities you enjoy. Switch your workout choices around if you like. You can walk the city streets, whirl around on your bike, or swim in the local pool. Participating in an exercise class that inspires you might be part of your regimen. Even if you don't think exercise is a smart idea, please try it. It will grow on you, I promise.

CHAPTER 5
Aerobic Exercise

There are many different types of exercise: one type might increase strength while a second might improve flexibility or balance; a third might be geared toward increased agility and coordination. All of these exercise types are important to help you maintain your independence. No one, after all, wants to live a long life if the last years are spent in bed relying on others to help you eat, go to the bathroom, or get dressed.

For example, leg strength is necessary to get out of a deep chair, to get off the toilet, and to help you get out of the bathtub. Arm strength is necessary to carry groceries and to lift things such as suitcases, grandchildren, and golf clubs. Without hip flexibility the length of strides you take while walking is shortened. Short steps lead to a shuffling gait, which is slower. When you walk slowly, your chances of falling are increased. Tight shoulders are injured more easily. Lack of flexibility in the rectus abdominis (large muscle reaching the entire length of the front of the stomach and intestines) leads to poor posture, digestive problems, and a protruding abdomen. Lack of balance can lead to falling, which is one of the major causes of injuries to older persons. Good balance is dependent upon strength and flexibility.

Another type of exercise that will strengthen the heart, lungs, and circulatory system is called aerobic (or endurance) exercise. A true aerobic exercise, one that elevates the heart rate and triggers the fat-burning metabolic rate, must be rhythmical, continuous, and sustained for a minimum of twenty minutes, three times a week in order to produce beneficial results (see benefits that follow). Activities such as walking, swimming, or biking are examples of aerobic exercise.

BENEFITS OF AEROBIC EXERCISE

- **Strengthens the heart.** During aerobic exercise, the heart muscle pumps more blood with each beat, resulting in a more efficient heart.

- **Improves circulation.** When the blood gets flowing, nutrients travel faster, oxygen gets to the muscles faster, and the exerciser has more energy.

- **Reduces blood pressure.** Aerobic exercise helps dilate (open) arteries. Naturally, open blood vessels do not have as much pressure as closed ones.

- **Increases HDL levels.** HDLs (high-density lipoproteins) are a type of cholesterol that is made up of small particles that easily pass through arteries. HDLs have protective effects. Having a high HDL level is good.

- **Reduces triglycerides.** Triglycerides are a type of fat that contributes to artery closure. Sustained rhythmical exercise reduces this type of fat in the blood.

- **Increases energy.** With an effective exercise program, the whole circulatory system works more efficiently, creating more energy.

- **Relieves tension.** Under stress, our body produces stress hormones. If stress hormones aren't put to good use, they will increase the heart rate and blood pressure. Unnecessary stress hormones quicken all our responses and create tension in the body. Aerobic exercise uses these produced-but-not-used stress hormones.

- **Improves sleep.** Regular aerobic exercise lessens tension in the muscles. With less tension, you'll sleep better. Exercise is certainly the preferred solution to sleepless nights—much better than using drugs, which can produce side effects.

- **Increases cell receptivity to insulin.** As we mature, bodily production of enzymes and hormones decreases. When less insulin is produced, there is a rise in blood sugar. To complicate things further, cells that normally use sugar from the blood can get sluggish and may not use the insulin or blood sugar that is available. This change in balance often results in diabetes. Many times, a good exercise and nutrition plan will correct the problem.

- **Increases bone density.** Our bones are not "dead" matter. They are constantly producing new red blood cells, moving calcium in and out of the blood stream, and making new bone cells. Aerobic exercise affects activity in the bone, helping to increase bone density.

- **Reduces body fat.** During the first twenty to thirty minutes of aerobic exercise, you will burn the energy that is already stored in the muscles. After that, you will burn fat. Even adding a one-mile walk a day to your daily routine can make a difference (you can lose about nine pounds a year). A good nutrition plan and an aerobic-exercise program can accelerate weight loss.

HEART-RATE TRAINING ZONES AND AEROBIC EXERCISE

Before beginning an aerobic workout, it is important to determine the intensity of training. The *heart-rate training zone* establishes the range of acceptable heartbeats per minute during aerobic exercise. Several formulas have been offered by exercise physiologists to calculate this range.

One of the most popular formulas is based on the theory that the average fastest human heartbeat (per minute) is 220. We know that as the body ages, its heart rate decreases by one beat each year. Therefore, you would subtract your age from 220 in order to establish your own *personal maximum heart rate.*

Once your personal maximum heart rate is established, your heart-rate zone can be formulated. This zone gives you the range of heartbeats (minimum to maximum) that you should achieve during a workout. For beneficial effects from exercise, your heart rate should reach at least 60 percent, but no more than 85 percent of your maximum heart rate during the most strenuous (working) phase of your aerobic workout.

Your goal should be to work within your heart-rate training zone. This will help produce the beneficial training effects listed on pages 66 and 67.

To establish your personal heart-rate training zone, simply use your age and follow the steps provided in the inset on page 68. If you prefer,

Establishing Your Heart-Rate Training Zone: A Simple Formula

Follow along as Evelyn, our model 70-year-old, determines her personal heart-rate training zone by following the steps below.

1. Evelyn subtracts 70 (her age) from 220 (average person's maximum heart rate during physical exercise).

        220 Maximum Heart Rate (average)
      − 70 Evelyn's Age
      150 Evelyn's Personal Maximum Heart Rate

2. Evelyn's heart rate should reach at least 60 percent of her personal maximum heart rate. Evelyn multiplies 150 (her maximum heart rate established in Step 1) by 60 percent. The resulting number is 90. During the working phase of her exercise session, Evelyn's heart should beat *at least* 90 times per minute.

        150 Evelyn's Personal Maximum Heart Rate
      x .60 Multiplier for establishing *Minimum* Training Zone
         90 Evelyn's *Minimum* Training-Zone Number

3. Evelyn's heart rate should not exceed 85 percent of her personal maximum heart rate. Evelyn multiplies 150 (her maximum heart rate established in Step 1) by 85 percent. The resulting number 127. During the working phase of her exercise session, Evelyn's heart should beat *no more than* 127 times per minute.

        150 Evelyn's Personal Maximum Heart Rate
      x .85 Multiplier for establishing *Maximum* Training Zone
       127 Evelyn's *Maximum* Training-Zone Number

By following these simple steps, Evelyn was able to establish her personal heart-rate training zone to be between 90−127. During the working phase of her exercise session, Evelyn's heart should beat between 90 and 127 beats per minute to achieve beneficial results (pages 66−67).

Table 5.1   Heart-Rate Zones

Age	Maximum Heart Rate	Heart-Rate Zone	Count in Ten Seconds
50−54	170	102−145	17−24
55−69	165	99−140	16−23
70−74	150	90−119	15−20
75−79	145	87−116	15−19
80−84	140	84−110	14−18
85−89	135	81−107	14−18
90−94	130	78−103	13−17
95−99	125	75−99	13−17
100	120	72−95	12−16

If you are on certain medications your heart rate may not be able to reach these levels. Check with your doctor before exercising.

however, use Table 5.1 to find the approximate range of your heart-rate training zone. Locate your age category in the left-hand column and move to the right until you locate your range. The last column establishes how many times your heart should beat for ten seconds (this number multiplied by six gives the number of beats per minute).

Let's assume you are between 80 and 84 years old. According to Table 5.1 you would have to exercise hard enough to get your heart rate up to 84 beats per minute (14 beats in ten seconds) but not higher than 110 beats per minute (18 beats in ten seconds).

MONITORING YOUR HEART RATE

A basic requirement of a good aerobic workout is the monitoring of your heart rate. Heart rates should be monitored several times during an aerobic activity. Your pre-exercise, *resting* heart rate should be taken before warming up. Monitoring your *exercising* heart rate during the working part of your exercise activity will ensure you are working within your heart-rate training zone (page 67). Finally, approximately three minutes into the cool-down phase of your workout, your heart rate should be monitored again. This is called your *recovery* heart rate. Your heart rate will return to normal more quickly as your aerobic fitness improves.

Finding Your Pulse

In order to check your heart rate, you must first be able to find your pulse. The best place to locate your pulse is at the wrist. Hold your hand with the palm up. Gently place the fingertips of your free hand on the wrist just under the thumb. You should feel your pulse beating beneath your fingertips. Starting at zero, count the number of beats you feel for ten seconds. Multiply this number by six for the number of beats per minute.

HOW TO DO AEROBIC EXERCISE

Three stages comprise a proper aerobic workout: the warm-up phase, the working phase, and the cool-down phase. All three stages are necessary to achieve beneficial effects (pages 66–67). Table 5.2 provides the proper warm-up, working, and cool-down times for each aerobic session.

How to Check Your Heart Rate

- *A good place to monitor your heart rate is at the wrist.*
- *Place your fingertips on the thumb side of your wrist. Roll your fingertips back just a little, pressing firmly until you feel a pulsation.*
- *Count the number of pulsations you feel for ten seconds.*
- *Multiply by six to get the count for one minute. (There are 6 ten-second periods in one minute.)*

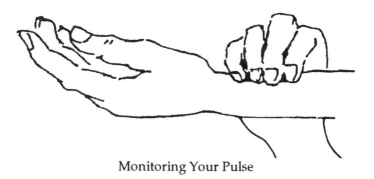

Monitoring Your Pulse

The Warm-Up

Most of our body's blood rests in the torso area, near our vital organs. During exercise, the blood must shift from this area to the working area of the body. This shift should be done slowly. If, for example, you have decided to take a walk, start slowly and build up speed as you go. This will give the circulatory system time to adjust and to move the needed extra blood and oxygen to the large muscles of the legs.

A five-minute warm-up period is usually sufficient. Perhaps you have chosen stationary cycling for your aerobic activity of the day. In this case, five minutes of pedaling at ten to fifteen miles per hour with no tension would be an appropriate warm-up. If walking is the aerobic activity you have choosen, five minutes of slow walking on a flat surface is considered an appropriate warm-up before gradually building up speed.

Before accelerating your exercise, take your pulse (page 70) to verify that you are in your training zone (page 67). Training zones are measured by heartbeats per minute. In order for aerobic exercise to be beneficial, the heartbeats per minute must be elevated above normal readings.

Never leap into a heavy routine or exercise program without giving your body a hint of what's coming. Always warm up, and remember: easy does it. You know that you are warmed up if your heart rate is at the lowest level of your training zone.

The Working Phase

Once you have warmed up, you are ready to begin the exercise portion of your aerobic workout. Remember that you can do any exercise that is rhythmical and continuous such as walking, biking, or swimming. I suggest that you begin with ten minutes of activity and when you are able, add one minute to each session until you can exercise a minimum of twenty-minutes. Remember that your warm-up and cool-down times should not be included in the twenty-minute working phase.

The Cool-Down

One of the most important phases of any exercise program is the cool-down period. When you exercise the large muscles, such as those in the legs, a large amount of blood is moved to these exercising muscles. Heart rate, blood pressure, and respiration are also increased.

The cool-down period allows all these body processes to slowly return to normal. Similar to the warm-up stage before starting to exercise, the best way to cool down is to simply slow down the activity you are doing. Five minutes of slower exercise is usually enough. You have officially cooled down when your heart rate falls below that of your training zone.

Table 5.2   Aerobic Exercise Program

Choose from the following suggested endurance activities for your aerobic workout: walking, swimming, rowing, hiking, and bicycling.

Session	Warm-Up	Exercise in Training Zone	Cool-Down
1	5 minutes (slowly)	10 minutes	7 minutes
2	5 minutes	11 minutes	7 minutes
3	5 minutes	12 minutes	7 minutes
4	5 minutes	13 minutes	7 minutes
5	5 minutes	14 minutes	7 minutes
6	5 minutes	15 minutes	7 minutes
7	5 minutes	16 minutes	7 minutes
8	5 minutes	17 minutes	6 minutes
9	5 minutes	18 minutes	6 minutes
10	5 minutes	19 minutes	6 minutes
11	5 minutes	20 minutes	6 minutes
12	5 minutes	21 minutes	6 minutes
13	5 minutes	22 minutes	6 minutes
14	5 minutes	23 minutes	6 minutes
15	5 minutes	24 minutes	5 minutes
16	5 minutes	25 minutes	5 minutes
17	5 minutes	26 minutes	5 minutes
18	5 minutes	27 minutes	5 minutes
19	5 minutes	28 minutes	5 minutes
20	5 minutes	29 minutes	5 minutes
21	5 minutes	30 minutes	5 minutes

For Best Aerobic Results

For an aerobic activity to produce benefits, it must be vigorous and sustained. Use the word "FIT" as your handy reminder that the road to aerobic fitness requires three things:

"F" for FREQUENCY   *To be beneficial, aerobic exercise must take place three times a week to develop and maintain cardiovascular function, and four to six times a week if you want to lose weight.*

"I" for INTENSITY   *The heart is a muscle that needs to be exercised like any other muscle. This exercise must take place in the heart-rate training zone (page 67).*

" T" for TIME   *For aerobic benefits, you must exercise twenty to sixty minutes continuously: twenty minutes for cardiorespiratory fitness; forty-five to sixty minutes for weight loss.*

RULES OF THUMB

Now that you are fortified with the best intentions, here are a few rules of thumb to go by:

- *Always check with your doctor or health-care provider before beginning any exercise program.*
- If you are just beginning an aerobic-exercise program, monitor your pulse more often, perhaps every five minutes.
- After you get to know your own body pattern, monitor less often: at the end of the warm-up period, at the end of the exercise phase, and at the end of the cool-down period.
- Begin with five minutes of warm-ups, ten minutes of exercises (or whatever you can), and seven minutes of cooling-down exercises.
- Gradually add one minute to the exercise phase of your workout (keep

five-minute warm-ups and cool-downs) until you build up to twenty to sixty minutes.
- Listen to your body. Never push yourself until you become breathless. You should be able to talk to someone while exercising.

Stop exercising if you:

- Feel faint, lightheaded, or dizzy.
- Feel nauseous.
- Experience chest pain.
- Experience pain in arms, jaws, teeth, or ears.
- Experience a loss of coordination.
- Experience a dramatic change in heart rate.
- Find your pulse does not read below 120 beats per minute within five minutes after you have stopped exercising.

CHAPTER 6
Sit-Down Workout

Depending on your physical condition, the following exercises, done while sitting in a chair, may suit you best. These exercises are less strenuous than many of those found in the General Conditioning Workout (Chapter 7), so they may be the perfect place to start your "new you" program. Good results are sure to follow if you are diligent and follow a program with regularity. Even though these exercises employ a gentle approach, remember to *always check with your doctor or health-care provider before beginning any exercise program.*

The exercises found in the Sit-Down Workout can help you improve the strength and flexibility in your neck, shoulders, arms, hands, wrists, back, and chest. They can also help strengthen your abdomen, hips, legs, and feet. Even if you try just a few, you'll soon realize how effective these exercises can be.

It is important to begin with a proper chair that "fits you." This means that you should be able to keep your feet flat on the floor while sitting straight up in the chair. Select a balanced, sturdy chair without arms so that you will be able to move your arms freely.

Keeping all these things in mind, get ready. It is time for you to "sit down on the job!"

Exercises for the Neck

An agile neck helps you live life safely. If your neck is flexible, you can turn your head easily when you're driving; you can also look up and down the street more readily when trying to cross busy intersections. Neck exercises are also excellent for reducing the tension that tightens neck muscles.

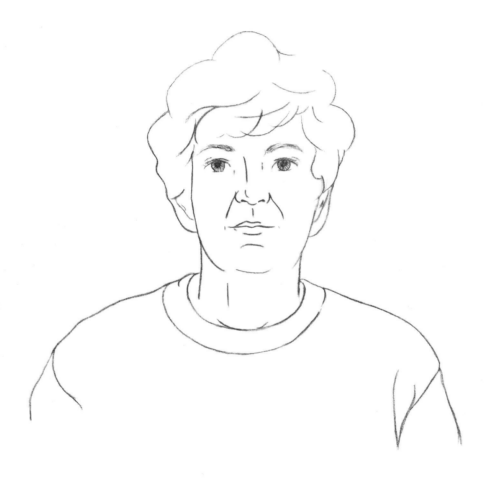

Head Rotation

STARTING POSITION: Sitting in a chair

DESIRED RESULT: Improvement in the flexibility of the neck muscles, which helps reduce pain from stiff, tense muscles and allows you to move your head more easily.

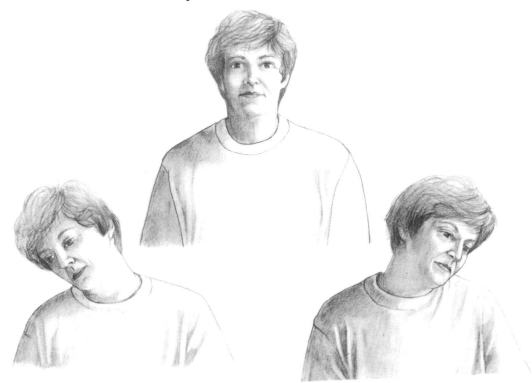

INSTRUCTIONS

1. Drop your head forward until your chin touches your chest.
2. Slowly roll your head in a com-
3. plete circle three times.
    Repeat three times going in the other direction.

- **You may notice that your neck is not very flexible. Don't get discouraged. You will see improvement if you stay with it.**

- **You may hear crunching sounds as you roll your head. While it may be noisy, nothing has been hurt. In fact, with regular exercise the sounds will probably go away.**

Looking Down

STARTING POSITION: Sitting in a chair

DESIRED RESULT: Improvement in the flexibility of the muscles found in the back of the neck, which helps reduce pain and increase motion.

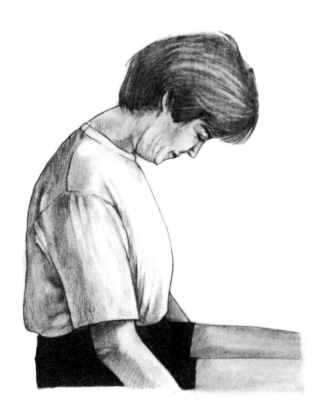

INSTRUCTIONS

1. Drop your head forward until your chin touches your chest, and you feel the stretch in the back of your neck.

2. Hold this position up to thirty seconds.

3. Do this exercise one time.

Looking Up

STARTING POSITION: Sitting in a chair

DESIRED RESULT: Improvement in the strength and flexibility of the muscles found in the front of the neck, which helps reduce pain and increase motion.

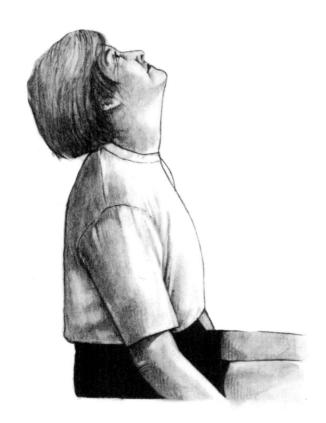

INSTRUCTIONS

1. Look up so your chin points to the ceiling.
2. Move your jaw in an exaggerated up-and-down "chewing" motion.
3. Repeat up to ten times.

Head Turns

STARTING POSITION: Sitting in a chair

DESIRED RESULT: Improvement in the flexibility of the neck muscles so you can easily turn your head from side to side. This will help you while driving or crossing the street.

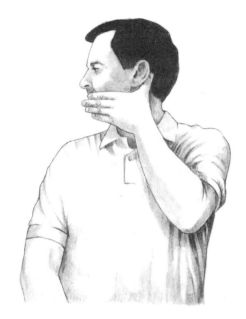

INSTRUCTIONS

1. Turn your head to the right until it lines up with your shoulder.
2. Place your left hand along the outside of your left jaw.
3. Gently push your head toward your shoulder.
4. Hold this postion up to thirty seconds.
5. Repeat on the other side.

It sounds like a simple instruction to "turn your head to the right until it lines up with your shoulder," but if you haven't been loosening up your neck muscles regularly, this simple action will be a challenge. Go easy on yourself at first, coaxing your head with gentle force. Soon, you'll notice that you've gained new ground on the head turn and will have more relaxed, agile neck muscles.

Exercises for the Shoulders and Arms

Rounded shoulders and a forward head lead to stooped posture. That's why the upper-body muscle groups are so important. Exercises that emphasize the backward motion of the arms and shoulders are particularly important for strengthening the upper chest and back muscles. Shoulder and arm exercises help develop the strength needed to lift groceries, golf clubs, suitcases, and grandchildren.

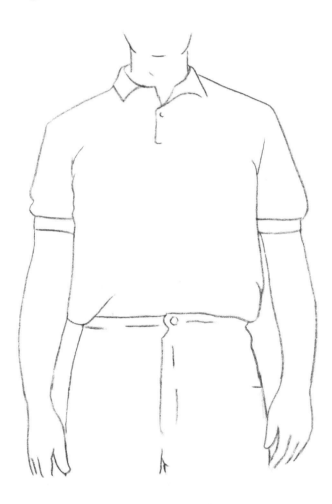

Shoulder Shrugs

STARTING POSITION: Sitting in a chair

DESIRED RESULT: Increased strength in the upper-shoulder muscles, which helps release tension and reduce shoulder pain.

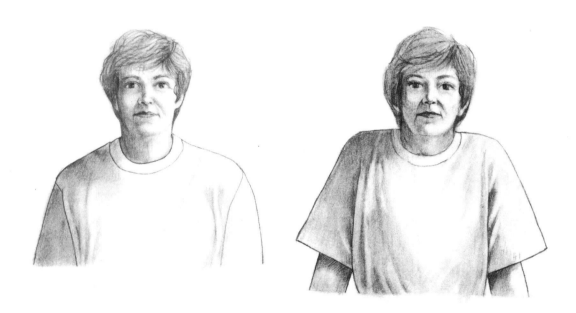

INSTRUCTIONS

1. Raise your shoulders up toward your ears, then bring them back
2. to the starting position. Repeat up to ten times.

Do not hold your shoulders in the raised position.

Shoulder Rotation

STARTING POSTION: Sitting in a chair

DESIRED RESULT: Tension relief in the shoulders and neck.

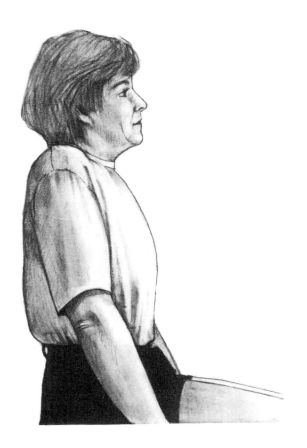
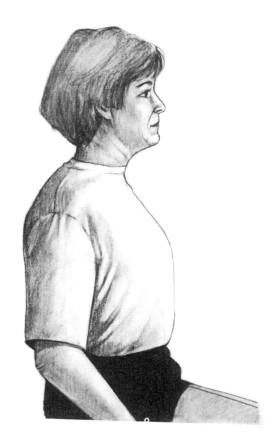

INSTRUCTIONS

1.   Roll your shoulders up toward your ears then down and back-   ward in a circular motion.
2.   Repeat up to ten times.

Only roll your shoulders backward since this direction encourages good posture.

Shoulder Stretch

STARTING POSITION: Sitting in a chair

DESIRED RESULT: Improvement in shoulder flexibility,which reduces the chance of injury and makes it easier to reach your back when zipping a dress or scratching an itch.

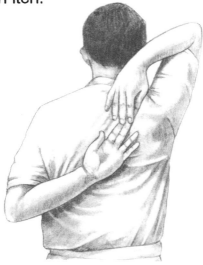

INSTRUCTIONS

1. Bring your right arm up and reach back over your right shoulder until your elbow points up and your fingertips touch your back. You'll feel stretching in the underside of your arm.

2. Bend your left arm behind your back and reach up until the fingers of your left hand meet the fingers of your right. Hold position up to thirty seconds.

3. Perform once on each side.

- **If you cannot make your hands meet behind your back, hold on to a towel, gradually moving your hands closer together.**

- **Many men have problems with this exercise. Women use this motion to zipper and button their dresses and to fasten their bras. Therefore, they are more flexible in the shoulders. Both men and women will find that it is easier to do this exercise on either their right or left side depending on whether they are right or left handed.**

Arm Circles

STARTING POSITION: Sitting in a chair

DESIRED RESULT: Increased strength in the arm and shoulder muscles, which helps when lifting things.

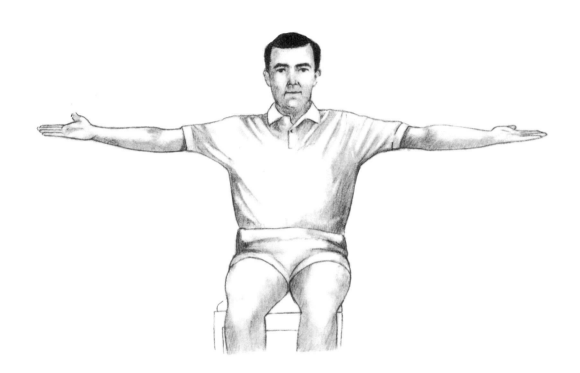

INSTRUCTIONS

1. Stretch your arms so they are out to your sides and shoulder high.
2. In a backward motion, with palms up, create circles with your extended arms.
3. Begin with 10 circles and gradually increase to 100.

Only roll your shoulders backward since this direction encourages good posture.

Overhead Arm Stretch

STARTING POSITION: Sitting in a chair

DESIRED RESULT: Increased flexibility of the shoulders and rib cage, which reduces the chance of injury and helps improve posture.

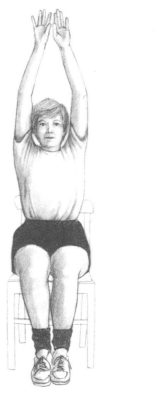 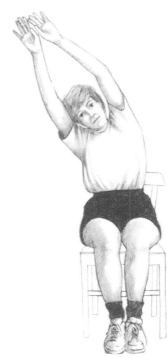

INSTRUCTIONS

1. Reach overhead with both arms until they are straight up and as close to your head as possible.
2. With your back firmly against the chair, lean to one side and then the other.
3. Repeat up to five times; gradually work up to ten.

To help prevent any injury during this exercise, make sure your back is against the chair for balance and support.

Random Arm Motions

STARTING POSITION: Sitting in a chair

DESIRED RESULT: Improvement in the coordination, strength, and flexibility in the arms and shoulders. This allows you to lift things more easily and reduces the chance of injury to these areas.

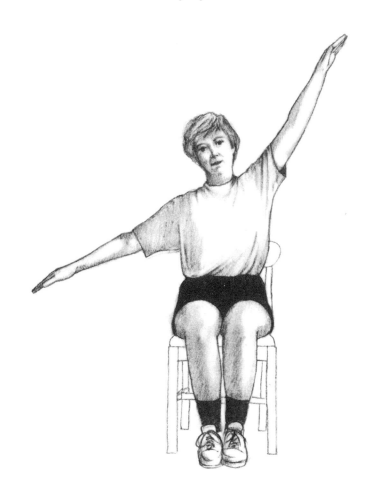

INSTRUCTIONS

1. Move your arms in random motions. Let your arms reach every way that they can, sometimes apart, sometimes together, out to the sides, up, and down.

2. Move your arms as quickly as you can.

3. Repeat up to ten times or more.

Large Arm Circles

STARTING POSITION: Sitting in a chair

DESIRED RESULT: Increased strength and range of motion in the arms and shoulders. This reduces pain and allows you to lift objects more easily.

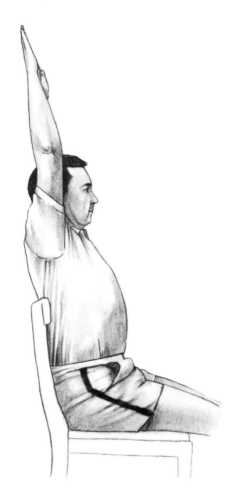

INSTRUCTIONS

1. Extend your arms straight out in front of you.
2. Make large circles at your sides with both arms. (Keep your arms as close to your head as possible as they come around.)
3. Repeat up to ten times in each direction.

Exercises for the Hands and Wrists

Hands and wrists need attention, too. Minimal effort can bring about wonderful results from the following hand and wrist exercises. A few minutes of attention in this area can improve strength and joint flexibility, resulting in hands that can write, sew, pick up change, and open tight lids with ease. Exercised hands also experience less pain from arthritis.

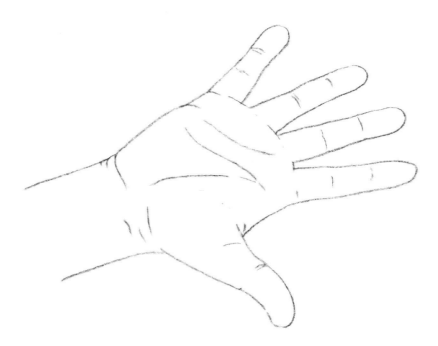

Finger Wiggling

STARTING POSITION: Sitting in a chair

DESIRED RESULT: Improvement in the flexibility and strength in the hands and fingers, making it easier to perform tasks such as sewing and picking up coins.

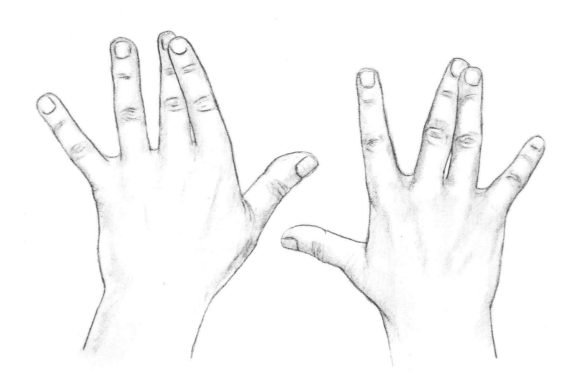

INSTRUCTIONS

1. With open hands, wiggle your fingers in all directions. You may choose to wiggle all your fingers together or each one separately.

2. Continue this motion up to thirty seconds.

Hand Stretch

STARTING POSITION: Sitting in a chair

DESIRED RESULT: Increased flexibility of the hands and fingers, which improves their range of motion and helps reduce pain.

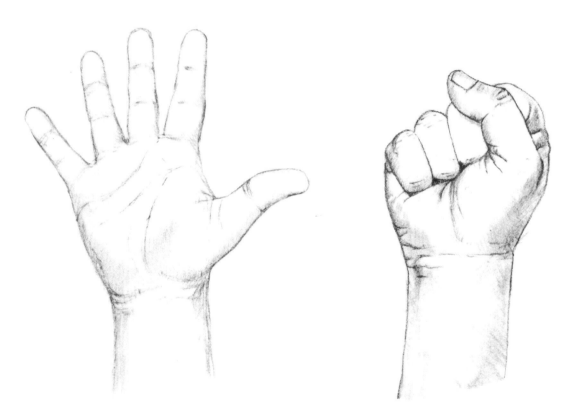

INSTRUCTIONS

1. Open your hands and stretch your fingers until you can feel a pull in the palms of your hands.
2. Make a fist.
3. Repeat up to ten times.

> **If you have arthritis in your hands, move slowly and emphasize the stretching part of this exercise.**

Thumb Stretch

STARTING POSITION: Sitting in a chair

DESIRED RESULT: Increased flexibility of the hands and thumbs, which improves their range of motion and helps reduce pain.

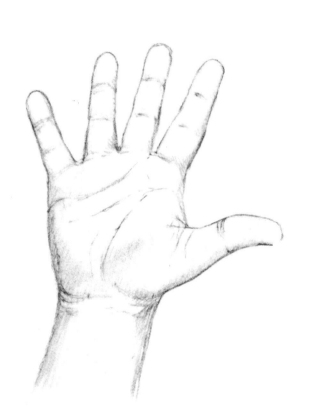 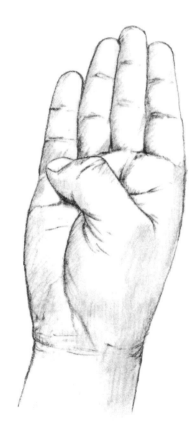

INSTRUCTIONS

1. With your fingers together, bring your thumb across the palm of your hand until it touches the base of your small finger.
2. Return the thumb to the starting position and stretch all your fingers for ten counts.
3. Repeat up to ten times. (You can perform this exercise with both hands at the same time.)

Small-Finger Stretch

STARTING POSITION: Sitting in a chair

DESIRED RESULT: Increased flexibility of the hands and small fingers, which improves their range of motion and helps reduce pain.

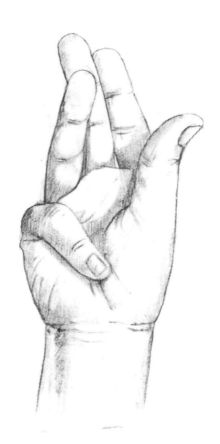

INSTRUCTIONS

1. With your fingers together, bring your small finger across the palm of your hand until it touches the base of your thumb.
2. Return your small finger to the starting position and stretch all your fingers for ten counts.
3. Repeat up to ten times. (You can perform this exercise with both hands at the same time.)

Middle-Finger Stretch 1

STARTING POSITION: Sitting in a chair

DESIRED RESULT: Increased flexibility of the hands and middle fingers, which improves their coordination. This helps when performing such tasks as handwriting and sewing.

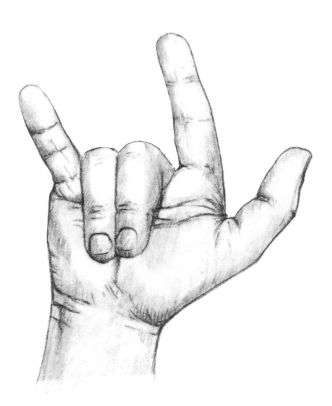

INSTRUCTIONS

1. With fingers extended straight out, bring your two middle fingers down to touch the palm of your hand. The two outside fingers should remain straight up.

2. Return your middle fingers to the starting position, then stretch all fingers for up to ten counts.

3. Repeat up to ten times. (You can do both hands at the same time.)

Middle-Finger Stretch 2

STARTING POSITION: Sitting in a chair

DESIRED RESULT: Increased flexibility of the hands and middle fingers, which improves their coordination.This helps when performing such tasks as handwriting and sewing.

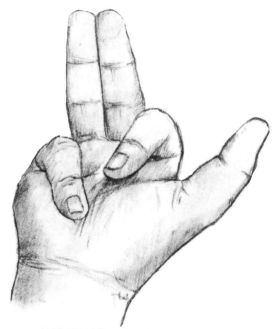

INSTRUCTIONS

1. With your fingers extended straight out, bring your two outside fingers down to touch the palm of your hand. The two inside fingers should remain straight up.

2. Return the outside fingers to the starting position, then stretch all the fingers for up to ten counts.

3. Repeat up to ten times. (You can do both hands at the same time.)

> **If you haven't done finger or hand exercises, you may find that your fingers don't like parting from one another. Don't worry, you can develop the coordination to move your fingers – both together and separately – with practice.**

Alternating Finger Stretch

STARTING POSITION: Sitting in a chair

DESIRED RESULT: Increased coordination, strength, and flexibility of the hands and fingers. This helps when performing fine motor-coordination tasks such as handwriting and picking up coins.

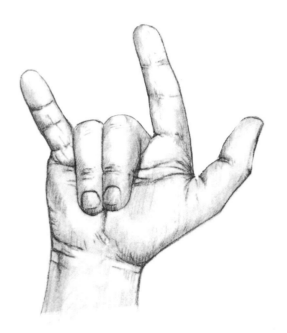
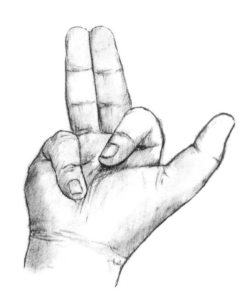

INSTRUCTIONS

1. Keeping your outside fingers up, bring your two middle fingers down to touch the palm of your hand.
2. Then switch, putting your outside fingers down and middle fingers up.
3. Alternate this motion as fast as you can up to ten times. (You can do both hands at the same time.)

Random Wrist Motions

STARTING POSITION: Sitting in a chair

DESIRED RESULT: Increased range of motion in the wrists, which improves mobility and helps reduce pain.

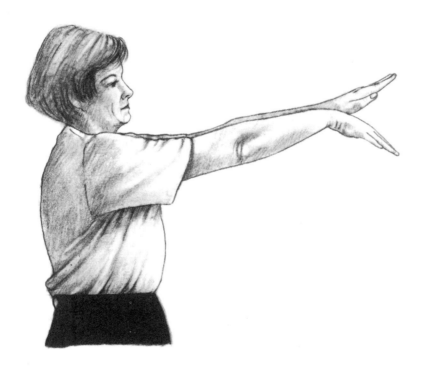

INSTRUCTIONS

1. With arms extended straight out in front of you, bend your hands at the wrists.
2. Move your wrists in all directions while keeping your fingers straight.
3. Repeat up to ten times in all directions.

Wrist Circling

STARTING POSITION: Sitting in a chair

DESIRED RESULT: Increased range of motion in the wrists, which improves mobility and helps reduce pain.

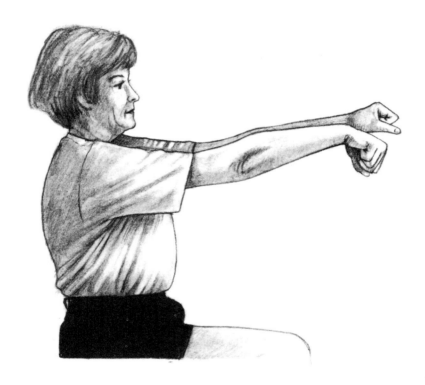

INSTRUCTIONS

1. Circle your wrists up to ten times in one direction and then the other.

2. Repeat up to ten times in each direction.

Exercises for the Torso, Upper Back, and Chest

As we age, our rib cage loses some of its flexibility. Torso exercises increase the flexibility of the muscles in the chest and at the sides of the body. This added flexibility makes breathing easier, improves posture, and allows turning and twisting without back injury. Exercises for the upper back and chest will help improve posture. When muscles tug and pull on bones, the bones become stronger. To prevent osteoporosis, exercises that work on the bones of the upper back are important.

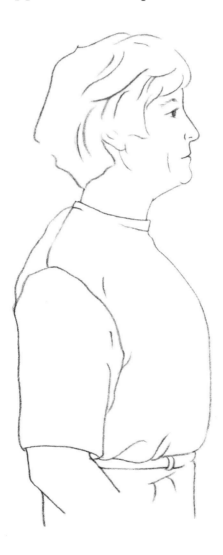

Upper-Back and Chest Stretch

STARTING POSITION: Sitting in a chair

DESIRED RESULT: Increased strength and flexibility of the upper back and chest, which encourages good posture.

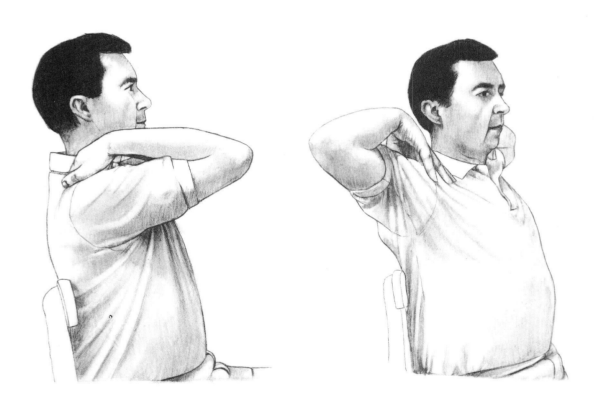

INSTRUCTIONS

1. Sit up straight and place your hands, palms down, on your shoulders.
2. Pull your arms toward the front of your body until your elbows meet. Keep your elbows as high as you can so that you feel the pull in your upper back.
3. Pull your arms back as far as you can so you feel stretching in your chest.
4. Repeat up to ten times.

Overhead-Arm and Torso Stretch

STARTING POSITION: Sitting in a chair

DESIRED RESULT: Increased flexibility of the arms, shoulders, and rib cage, which encourages good posture. Improved rib cage flexibility may also improve breathing.

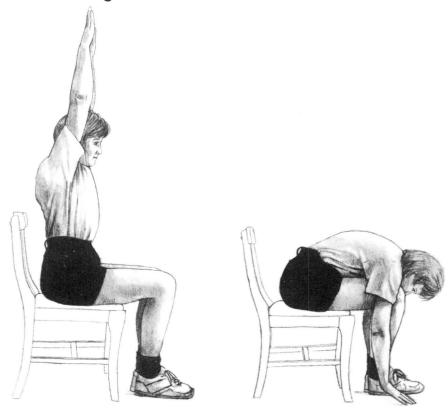

INSTRUCTIONS

1. Reach overhead with outstretched arms.
2. Pull your upper arms in so that they touch the sides of your head.
3. Clasp hands together and pull your arms up. (You'll feel a lifting in the shoulders, ribs, and waist.) While holding this position, take a deep breath and count to ten.
4. Exhale for ten counts while bending down and bringing your arms down to the floor.
5. Inhale and return to the starting position.
6. Repeat up to ten times.

Side Stretch

STARTING POSITION: Sitting in a chair

DESIRED RESULT: Increased strength and flexibility of the rib cage, and improved strength in the muscles found at the sides of your body. This helps improve breathing and promotes good posture.

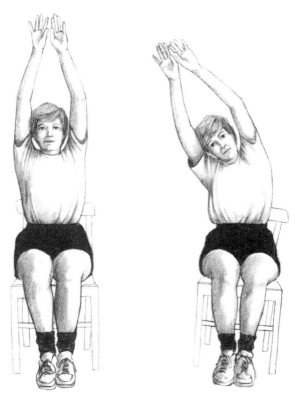

INSTRUCTIONS

1. While sitting up straight with your back against the chair, inhale and silently count to ten while raising your arms over your head.

2. Exhale for ten counts while leaning to one side.

3. Hold that position for ten counts.

4. Return to the original position.

5. Repeat up to ten times on each side.

To help prevent any injury during this exercise, make sure your back is against the chair when leaning to the side.

Rib Stretch

STARTING POSITION: Sitting in a chair

DESIRED RESULT: Increased strength and flexibility of the rib cage and torso, which helps improve breathing and promotes good posture .

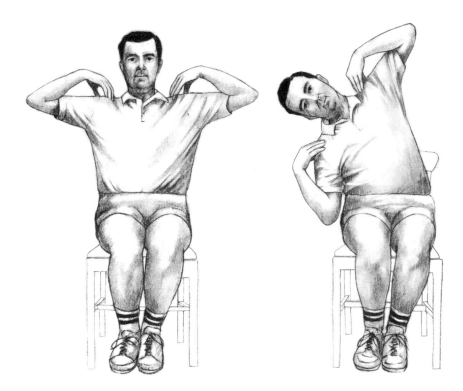

INSTRUCTIONS

1. Sit up straight and place your hands, palms down, on your shoulders.
2. Lean to the right until your right elbow touches the chair seat.
3. Lift your left elbow as high as you can. This action will stretch the side of your body.
4. Return to a sitting position and repeat on the other side.
5. Repeat ten times slowly and then ten times as fast as you can.

To help prevent any injury during this exercise, make sure your back is against the chair when leaning to the side.

Trunk Twister

STARTING POSITION: Sitting in a chair

DESIRED RESULT: Increased strength and flexibility of the muscles in the middle and lower back, which helps reduce the chance of injury to your back.

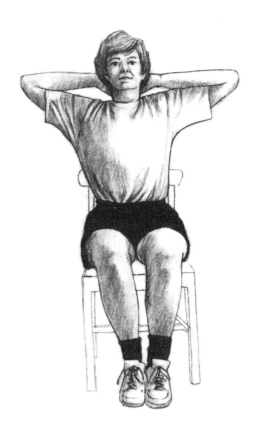 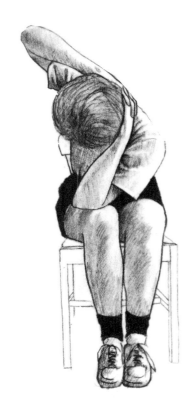

INSTRUCTIONS

1. Sit up straight in the chair and clasp your hands behind your neck.
2. Twist down so that your right elbow touches the outside of your left knee.
3. While bent over, look up at the elbow that is pointing to the ceiling and hold this position up to thirty seconds.
4. Do only one time on each side.

Exercises for the Abdomen

Strong abdominal muscles are a must for good posture, for keeping the abdominal organs in their proper positions, and for preventing or alleviating lower-back problems. These muscles are generally weak and may take a long time to improve. Be positive. Keep going. Every time you exercise, you are strengthening these muscles. Be careful not to jerk or strain.

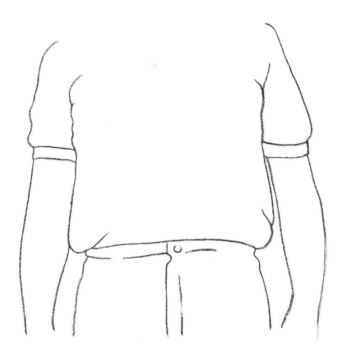

Abdominal Pushes

STARTING POSITION: Sitting in a chair

DESIRED RESULT: Increased strength in the abdominal muscles, which helps prevent back injuries.

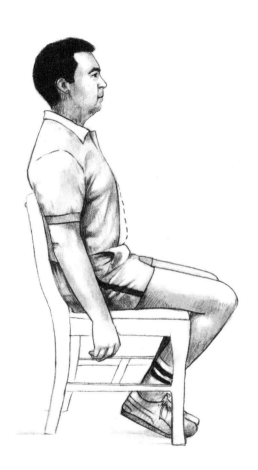

INSTRUCTIONS

1. Push your abdominal muscles in and out as hard as you can.

2. Repeat up to ten times or more.

Abdominal Hand Pushes

STARTING POSITION: Sitting in a chair

DESIRED RESULT: Increased strength in the abdominal muscles, which helps prevent back injuries.

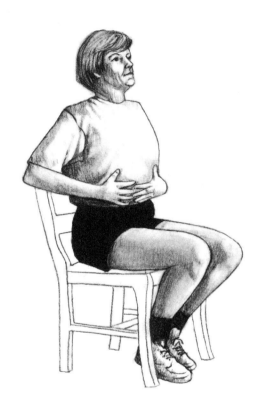

INSTRUCTIONS

1. Place the palms of your hands on your abdomen.
2. Press your abdominal muscles against your hands and breathe out. You will feel the muscles tighten against your hands. Relax the muscles.
3. Repeat at least ten times.

> **Make sure you breathe while doing this exercise. Holding your breath could increase your blood pressure.**

Leg Lifts

STARTING POSITION: Sitting in a chair

DESIRED RESULT: Increased strength in the upper legs and abdomen, which helps when doing such things as getting out of the bathtub and getting up off the floor.

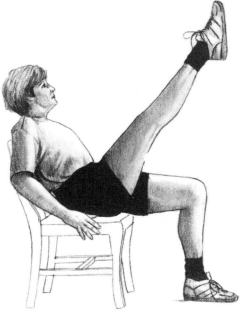

INSTRUCTIONS

1. Sit on the edge of the chair with your upper back leaning against the chair back.
2. Hang on to the sides of the seat. Straighten one leg and lift it as high as you can. Return the leg to the starting position and repeat with the other leg.
3. Repeat up to ten times with each leg.

- **Make sure you breathe while doing this exercise. Holding your breath could increase your blood pressure.**

- **If you have back problems, sit with your entire back against the chair back. Try to lift your thigh off the chair.**

- **A more advanced variation would be to lift both legs at the same time. Start with three lifts and increase up to ten.**

Ins and Outs

STARTING POSITION: Sitting in a chair

DESIRED RESULT: Increased strength in the abdominal and upper-leg muscles, which helps reduce the chance of lower-back injury.

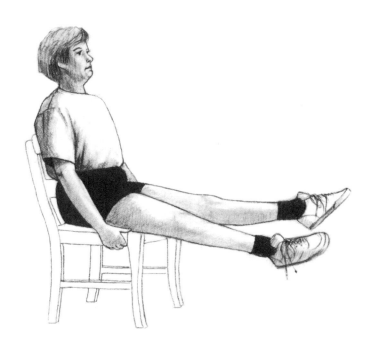

INSTRUCTIONS

1. Hold on to the sides of the chair and strengthen both legs up in the air until your feet are even with the chair seat.
2. Keep your legs straight and move them apart as far as you can. Your legs will dangle in the air forming a "v" pattern.
3. Bring your legs back together without allowing your feet to rest on the floor.
4. Repeat up to ten times.

Exercises for the Hips and Legs

If a quality life is what you desire, you must be independent in doing things for yourself. You must be able to walk, climb stairs, bend down, get up, and do a certain amount of lifting. All of these moves are dependent on strong leg and hip muscles. Having strong, flexible hips will enable you to take longer steps and walk faster, which may help prevent falling. Putting force on the hips also helps increase the strength of the hip bones.

One of the best ways to improve hip and leg muscles is by doing a lot of walking. Muscles respond to stress. If you have trouble walking, then walking is exactly what you should do to improve the situation. The following exercises are excellent examples of hip and leg strengtheners.

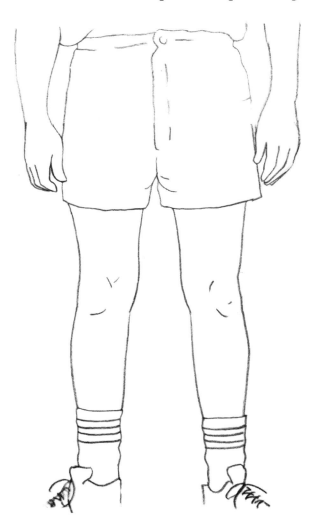

Hip Stretch

STARTING POSITION: Sitting in a chair

DESIRED RESULT: Increased flexibilty of the hips, which allows you to walk better.

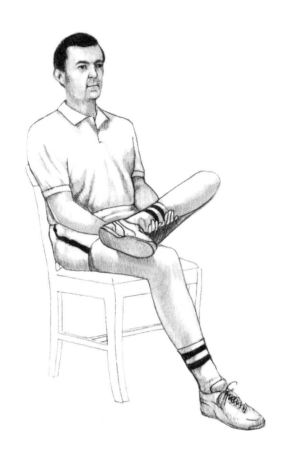

INSTRUCTIONS

1. Sitting up straight, bend your right leg at the knee and place your right ankle on top of your left thigh.
2. Grab hold of your right ankle and calf with both of your hands and pull until your foot is as close to your chest as possible.
3. The movement of the right leg pulling up will create a stretch in the right hip. Hold this stretch up to thirty seconds.
4. Do this exercise one time with each leg.

Knee-to-Chest Stretch

STARTING POSITION: Sitting in a chair

DESIRED RESULT: Increased flexibility of the lower back.

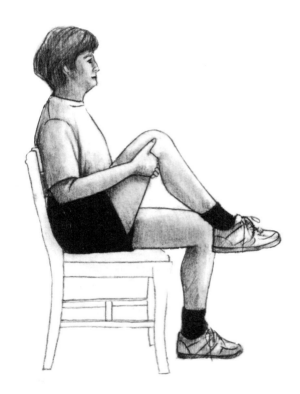

INSTRUCTIONS

1. Sit up straight with both feet flat on the floor.
2. Clasp your hands under one thigh and pull your knee toward your chest. Hold for ten counts.
3. Return your leg to the starting position.
4. Repeat up to ten times with each leg .

Chair Jogging

STARTING POSITION: Sitting in a chair

DESIRED RESULT: Increased strength and flexibility of the legs, which makes walking easier.

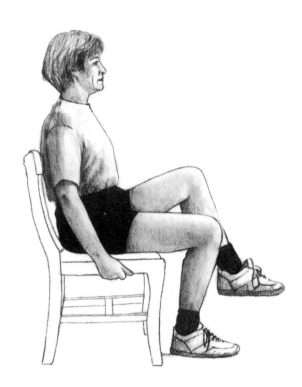

INSTRUCTIONS

1. Move your legs up and down as if you are jogging as fast as you can. If needed, hang on to the chair to steady yourself.

2. Repeat ten times or more.

For an even better workout, bring your knees up to your chest when "jogging."

Upper-Leg Strengthener

STARTING POSITION: Sitting in a chair

DESIRED RESULT: Increased strength in the upper thighs. This helps when performing such movements as getting out of the back seat of a car or a deep chair and when getting up off the floor.

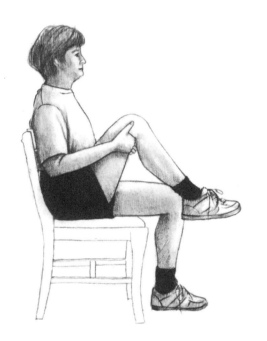
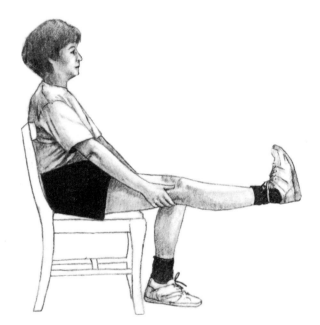

INSTRUCTIONS

1. Clasp your hands under one thigh and pull it to your chest.
2. Straighten your leg out in front of you. Your heel should be as high as the chair seat.
3. Bring your thigh back to your chest.
4. Repeat up to ten times before returning your foot to the floor.
5. Repeat with the other thigh.

Straight-Leg Hold

STARTING POSITION: Sitting in a chair

DESIRED RESULT: Increased strength in the upper legs, which helps when climbing stairs, bending down, and getting out of deep chairs.

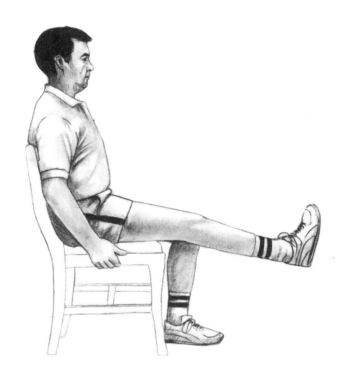

INSTRUCTIONS

1.   Holding on to the sides of the chair, sit up straight with both feet flat on the foor.
2.   Extend your right leg straight out in front of you, making sure your leg is as high as the seat of the chair. Hold for up to ten counts without holding your breath.
3.   Return to the original position.
4.   Repeat up to ten times with each leg.

Straight-Leg Lifts

STARTING POSITION: Sitting in a chair

DESIRED RESULT: Increased strength in the upper legs, which helps when climbing stairs, bending down, and getting out of deep chairs.

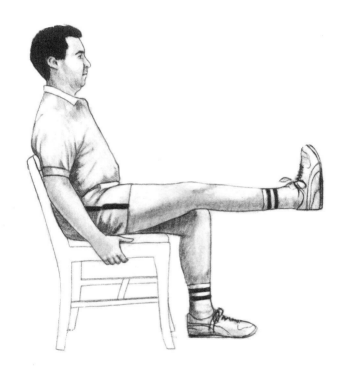

INSTRUCTIONS

1. Holding on to the sides of the chair, sit up straight with both feet flat on floor.
2. Extend your right leg straight out in front of you, making sure it is as high as the seat of the chair.
3. Lift your leg about six inches off the chair.
4. Repeat lift up to ten times, then return leg to the starting position.
5. Repeat with the other leg.

Side Kicks

STARTING POSITION: Sitting in a chair

DESIRED RESULT: Increased strength and flexibility of the legs and hips, which will help you walk better.

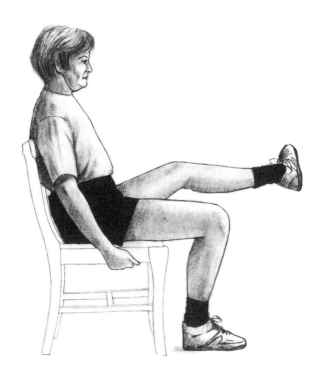

INSTRUCTIONS

1. Sit up straight with both feet flat on the floor.
2. Extend your right leg straight in front of you, making sure it is as high as the seat of the chair.
3. Turn your right foot out to the right.
4. Bend your knee and move your leg to the right side, straightening your leg as you move it. Continue bending and straightening up to ten times.
5. Return your leg to the starting position.
6. Repeat up to ten times on each side.

Hip Lifts

STARTING POSITION: Sitting in a chair

DESIRED RESULT: Increased flexibility of the hips, which makes walking easier and reduces the chance of injury.

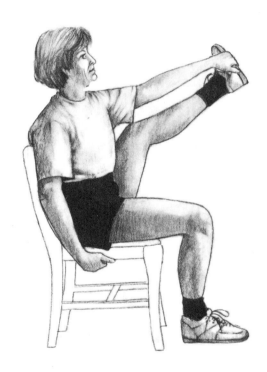

INSTRUCTIONS

1. Sitting up straight, grab the sole of your right foot with your right hand and straighten your leg out as best you can.

2. Hold this stretch up to thirty seconds.

3. Do this exercise one time with each leg.

Exercises for the Feet and Ankles

We depend on our feet to get us around, but they are often ignored unless we feel pain or discomfort when walking. Foot exercises may seem odd at first, but they are an important part of foot care. These exercises strengthen the toes and feet promoting good balance.

Characteristically, diabetics have poor circulation in the lower extremities. Therefore, good foot care is especially important for those with diabetes.

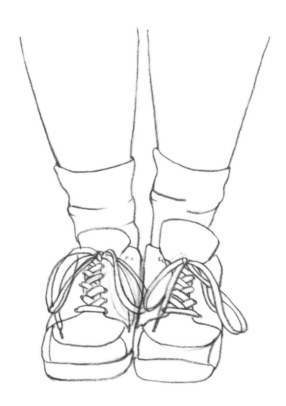

Toe Wiggling

STARTING POSITION: Sitting in a chair

DESIRED RESULT: Increased flexibility of the toes and feet, which promotes good balance.

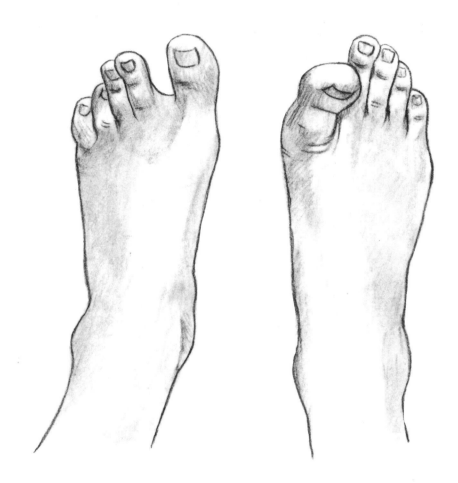

INSTRUCTIONS

1.   Remove your shoes and wiggle your toes.

2.   Do this up to thirty seconds.

Toe Stretches

STARTING POSITION: Sitting in a chair

DESIRED RESULT: Increased flexibility of the toes and feet, which promotes good balance.

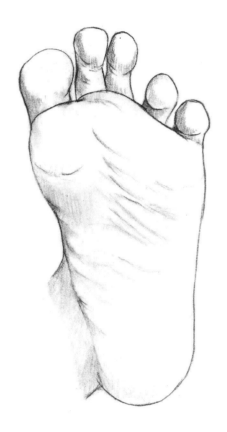
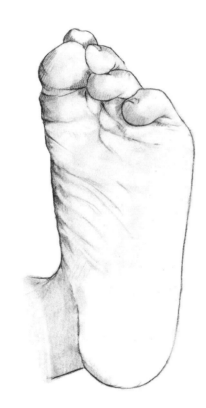

INSTRUCTIONS

1. Remove your shoes and stretch your toes as far apart as you can.
2. Relax the stretch and curl your toes under.
3. Continue stretching and curling up to ten times. (You can perform this exercise with both feet at the same time.)

Toe Lifts

STARTING POSITION: Sitting in a chair

DESIRED RESULT: Increased strength and flexibility of the feet, which promotes good balance.

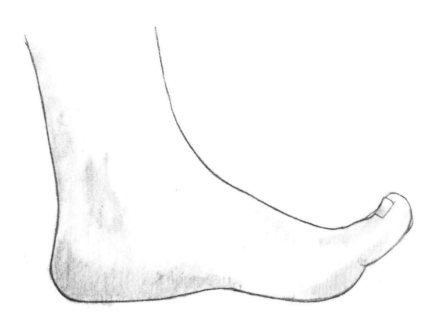

INSTRUCTIONS

1. Remove your shoes and put your feet flat on the floor.
2. Keep the soles of your feet on the floor and lift all your toes as high as you can.
3. Do this up to ten times. (You can perform this exercise with both feet at the same time.)

Big-Toe Lifts

STARTING POSITION: Sitting in a chair

DESIRED RESULT: Increased strength and flexibility of the big toes, which promote good balance.

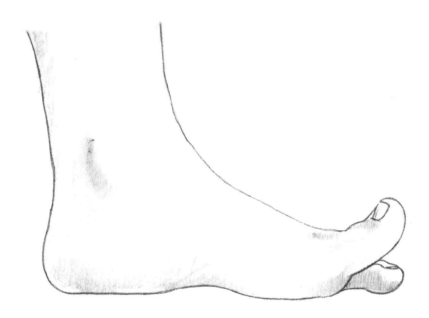

INSTRUCTIONS

1. Remove your shoes and put your feet flat on the floor.
2. Keep the soles of your feet on the floor; lift your big toe only.
3. Do this up to ten times. (You can perform this exercise with both feet at the same time.)

If you have a problem lifting your big toe only, hold the small toes down with your fingers.

Small-Toe Lifts

STARTING POSITION: Sitting in a chair

DESIRED RESULT: Increased strength and flexibility of the feet and toes, which promotes good balance.

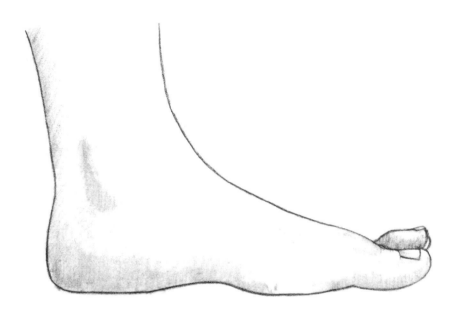

INSTRUCTIONS

1. Remove your shoes and put your feet flat on the floor.
2. Keep the soles of your feet on the floor and lift your small toes only.
3. Do this up to ten times. (You can perform this exercise with both feet at the same time.)

If you have a problem lifting your small toes only, hold the big toe down with your fingers.

Foot Lifts

STARTING POSITION:　Sitting in a chair

DESIRED RESULT:　Increased muscle strength in the lower legs and ankles, which promotes good balance.

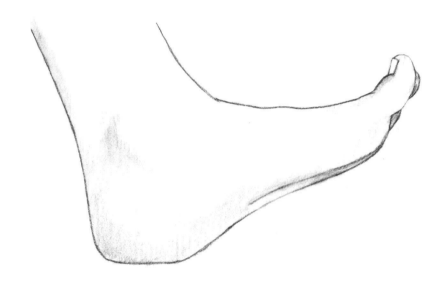

INSTRUCTIONS

1.　Keeping your heels on the floor, lift up the soles of your feet.
2.　Repeat up to ten times. (You can perform this exercise with both feet at the same time.)

Foot lifts are harder to do when your feet are close to the legs of the chair.

Ankle Rolls

STARTING POSITION: Sitting in a chair

DESIRED RESULT: Increased strength and flexibility of the feet, which promotes good balance.

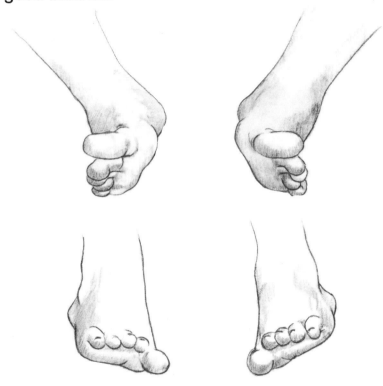

INSTRUCTIONS

1. Roll your feet to the inside edges   2.   Repeat up to ten times.
    and then to the outside edges.

Congratulations! The chair exercises for the Sit-Down Workout have been completed, but your session is not over yet. I strongly recommend that you follow your workout with some (or all) of the stretching exercises in Chapter 8. These stretches can be done while standing, sitting, or lying down.

Finally, stand up (think of this as giving yourself a standing ovation), and complete the following final exercise, which will enhance your balance.

Balancing Act

STARTING POSITION: Standing up

DESIRED RESULT: Improvement in balance.

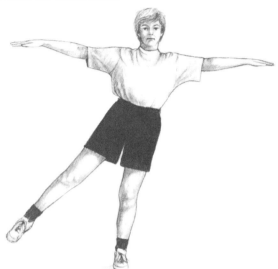

INSTRUCTIONS

1. Stand with your feet comfortably apart and extend your arms straight out to the sides for balance.
2. Lift your right foot off the floor. You can lift it to the side or the front. You can bend your knee or keep your leg straight, whichever is most comfortable for you.
3. Hold for up to ten counts.
4. Bring your foot back down and repeat with your left leg.
5. For a more advanced version, you can lift your foot, hold for ten seconds, and move from the front to the side position. Count for another ten seconds before moving your foot back to the original position.

- **If you are just starting, you may want to rest a free hand lightly on the back of a chair to steady yourself.**
- **It is easier to maintain your balance if you tighten your supporting leg and buttocks while your other foot is in the air.**
- **Pick a spot on the floor and focus on it while balancing.**
- **This exercise will become easier with practice.**

CHAPTER 7
General Conditioning Workout

The General Conditioning Workout is designed for men and women of any age who are in general good health. (This workout certainly gives the college students who visit my class a "run for their money.") As with the Sit-Down Workout, presented in Chapter 6, the General Conditioning Workout is geared toward developing and maintaining strength, flexibility, agility, balance, and coordination. After only a few weeks of doing these exercises, you will notice an increase in your range of motion. (Range of motion refers to the normal amount of motion a joint can perform without causing injury.) Continued exercise also improves reaction time, which is especially important if you drive.

The General Conditioning Workout provides exercises for every part of the body, from head to toe. Some exercises are the same as those found in the Sit-Down Workout, others are similar but harder to do, and others are unique to this workout.

For comfort and safety, be sure to use a mat when performing the exercises in this chapter. Never exercise on a hard floor! And most important: *remember to consult your doctor or health-care provider before beginning any exercise program.*

Exercises for the Neck

An agile neck helps you live life safely. If your neck is flexible, you can turn your head easily when you're driving; you can also look up and down the street more readily when trying to cross busy intersections. Neck exercises are also excellent for reducing the tension that tightens neck muscles.

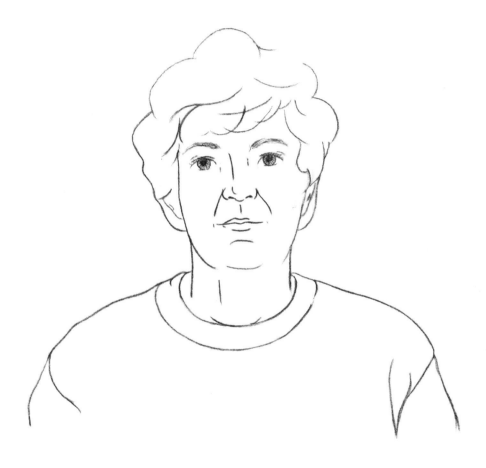

Head Rotation

STARTING POSITION: Standing

DESIRED RESULT: Improvement in the flexibility of the neck muscles, which helps reduce pain from stiff, tense muscles and allows you to move your head more easily.

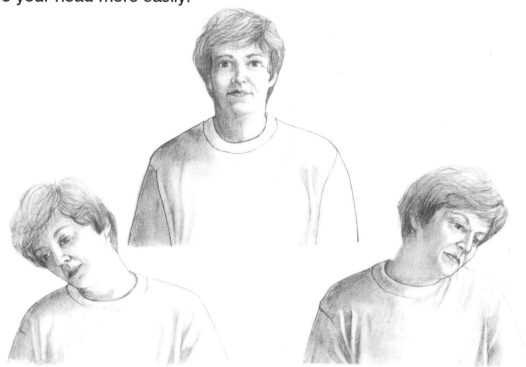

INSTRUCTIONS

1. Drop your head forward until your chin touches your chest.
2. Slowly roll your head in a complete circle three times.
3. Repeat three times going in the other direction.

- **You may notice that your neck is not very flexible. Don't get discouraged. You will see improvement if you stay with it.**

- **You may hear crunching sounds as you roll your head. While it may be noisy, nothing has been hurt. In fact, with regular exercise the sounds will probably go away.**

Looking Down

STARTING POSITION: Standing

DESIRED RESULT: Improvement in the flexibility of the muscles found in the back of the neck, which helps reduce pain and increase motion.

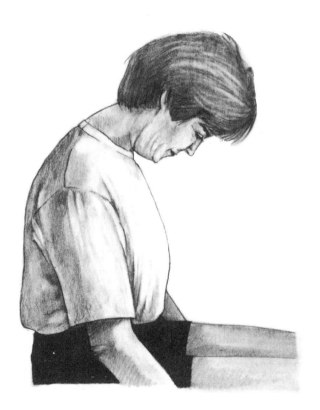

INSTRUCTIONS

1. Drop your head forward until your chin touches your chest and you feel the stretch in the back of your neck.

2. Hold this position up to thirty seconds.

3. Do this exercise one time.

Looking Up

STARTING POSITION: Standing

DESIRED RESULT: Improvement in the strength and flexibility of the muscles found in the front of the neck, which helps reduce pain and increase motion.

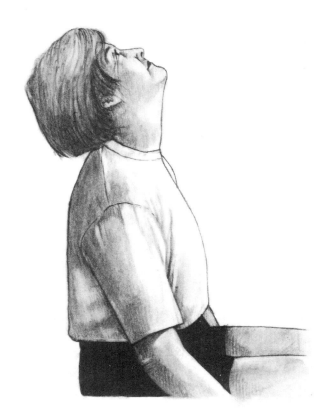

INSTRUCTIONS

1. Look up so your chin points to the ceiling.
2. Move your jaw in an exagger-ated up-and-down "chewing" motion.
3. Repeat up to ten times.

Head Turns

STARTING POSITION: Standing

DESIRED RESULT: Improvement in the flexibility of the neck muscles so you can easily turn your head from side to side. This will help you while driving or when crossing the street.

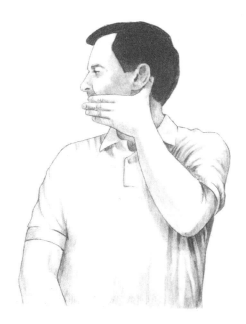

INSTRUCTIONS

1. Turn your head to the right until it lines up with your shoulder.

2. Place your left hand along the outside of your left jaw.

3. Gently push your head toward your shoulder.

4. Hold this position up to thirty seconds.

5. Repeat on the other side.

It sounds like a simple instruction to "turn your head to the right until it lines up with your shoulder," but if you haven't been loosening up your neck muscles regularly, this simple action will be a challenge. Go easy on yourself at first, coaxing your head with gentle force. Soon, you'll notice that you've gained new ground on the head turn and will have more relaxed, agile neck muscles.

Exercises for the Shoulders and Arms

Rounded shoulders and a forward head lead to stooped posture. That's why the upper-body muscle groups are so important. Exercises that emphasize the backward motion of the arms and shoulders are particularly important for strengthening the upper chest and back muscles. Shoulder and arm exercises help develop the strength needed to lift groceries, golf clubs, suitcases, and grandchildren.

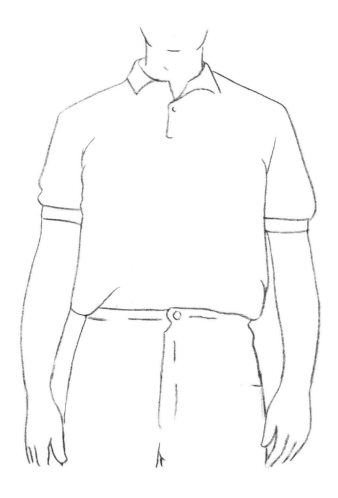

Shoulder Shrugs

STARTING POSITION: Standing

DESIRED RESULT: Increased strength in the upper-shoulder muscles, which helps release tension and reduce shoulder pain.

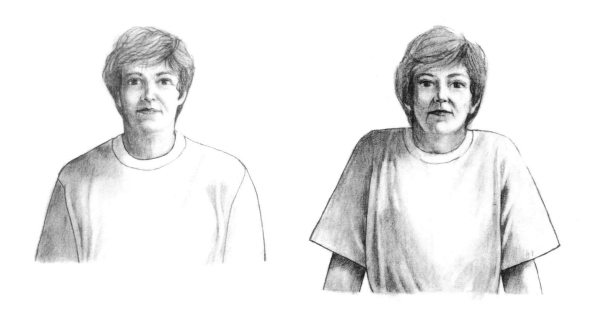

INSTRUCTIONS

1. Raise your shoulders up toward your ears, then bring them back to the starting position.
2. Repeat up to ten times.

Do not hold your shoulders in the raised position.

Shoulder Rotation

STARTING POSITION: Standing

DESIRED RESULT: Tension relief in the shoulders and neck.

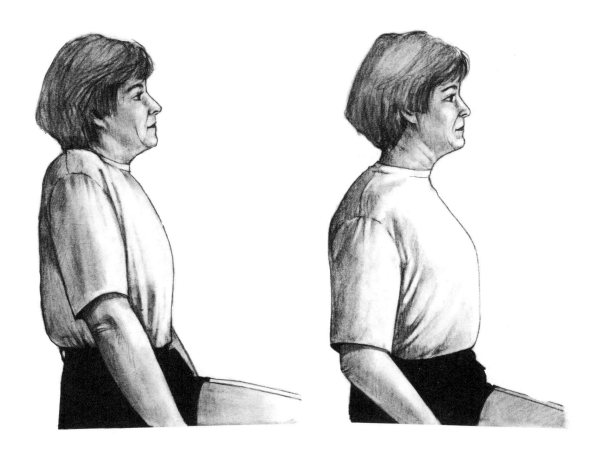

INSTRUCTIONS

1. Roll your shoulders up toward your ears then down and back-
2. ward in a circular motion. Repeat up to ten times.

Only roll your shoulders backward since this direction encourages good posture.

Push-Ups

STARTING POSITION: On hands and knees (on mat)

DESIRED RESULT: Increased arm and shoulder strength, which helps when lifting heavy objects.

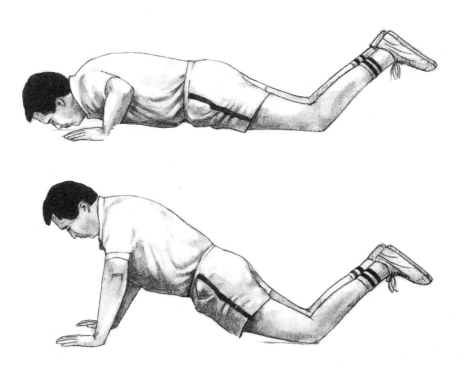

INSTRUCTIONS

1. Position yourself on your hands and knees on a mat.
2. Place your hands directly under your shoulders and bend your legs so that your lower legs are lifted in the air. Keep your torso straight.
3. Bend your elbows and lower yourself to the floor.
4. Return to the starting position.
5. Repeat up to ten times.

Shoulder Stretch 1

STARTING POSITION: Standing

DESIRED RESULT: Improvement in shoulder flexibility, which reduces the chance of injury and makes it easier to reach your back when zipping a dress or scratching an itch.

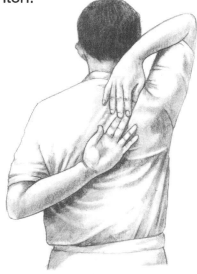

INSTRUCTIONS

1. Bring your right arm up and reach back over your right shoulder until your elbow points up and your fingertips touch your back. You'll feel stretching in the underside of your arm.

2. Bend your left arm behind your back and reach up until the fingers of your left hand meet the fingers of your right. Hold position up to thirty seconds.

3. Perform once on each side.

- **If you cannot make your hands meet behind your back, hold on to a towel, gradually moving your hands closer together.**

- **Many men have problems with this exercise. Women use this motion to zipper and button their dresses and to fasten their bras. Therefore they are more flexible in the shoulders. Both men and women will find that it is easier to do this exercise on either their right or left side depending upon whether they are right or left handed.**

Shoulder Stretch 2

STARTING POSITION: Sitting on floor (on mat)

DESIRED RESULT: Improvement in shoulder flexibility, which increases range of motion.

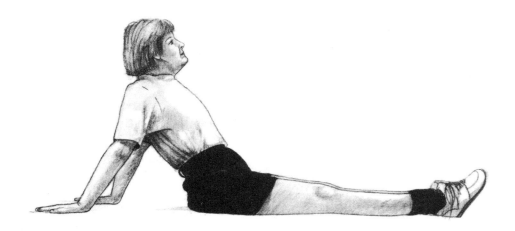

INSTRUCTIONS

1. Sit on the floor and straighten out your arms behind your shoulders. Rest the palms of your hands on the floor.
2. Scoot forward. You will feel your shoulder blades coming to-

gether in the center of your back. You will also feel a stretch in your shoulders and arms.
3. Hold this position up to thirty seconds.
4. Do this exercise one time.

Arm Circles

STARTING POSITION: Standing

DESIRED RESULT: Increased strength in the arm and shoulder muscles, which helps when lifting things.

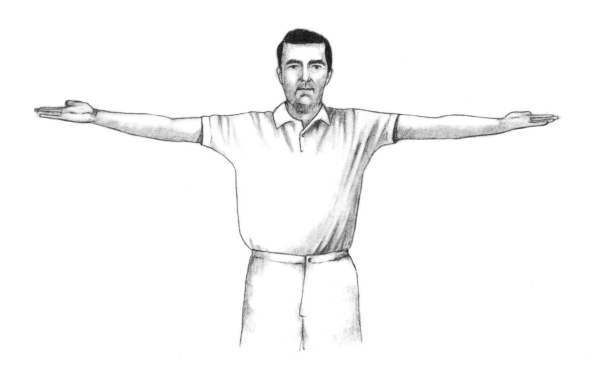

INSTRUCTIONS

1. Stretch your arms so they are out to your sides and shoulder high.
2. In a backward motion, with palms up, create circles with your extended arms.
3. Begin with 10 circles and gradually increase to 100.

Only roll your shoulders backward since this direction encourages good posture.

Large Arm Circles

STARTING POSITION: Standing

DESIRED RESULT: Increased strength and range of motion in the arms and shoulders. This reduces pain and allows you to lift objects more easily.

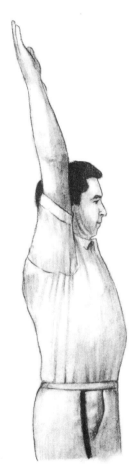

INSTRUCTIONS

1. Extend your arms straight out in front of you.
2. Make large circles at your sides with both arms. (Keep your arms as close to your head as possible as they come around.)
3. Repeat up to ten times in each direction.

Arm Crossing

STARTING POSITION: Standing

DESIRED RESULT: Increased strength in arm and shoulder muscles, which helps when lifting things.

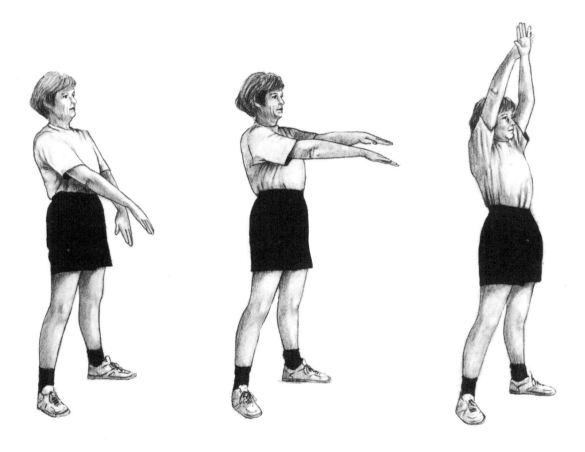

INSTRUCTIONS

1. Straighten both arms in front of you, then lower them until your fingers point to the floor.
2. Cross your arms, first over and then under each other.
3. Repeat ten times.
4. Raise your arms until they are shoulder high. Repeat the cross-over motion ten times.
5. Raise your extended arms over-head and repeat the cross-over motion ten times.

Exercises for the Hands and Wrists

Hands and wrists need attention, too. Minimal effort can bring about wonderful results from the following hand and wrist exercises. A few minutes of attention in this area can improve strength and joint flexibility, resulting in hands that can write, sew, pick up change, and open tight lids with ease. Exercised hands also experience less pain from arthritis.

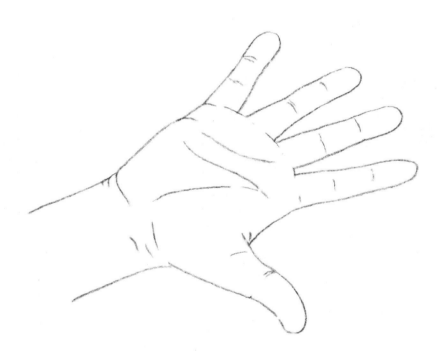

Finger Wiggling

STARTING POSITION: Standing

DESIRED RESULT: Improvement in the flexibility and strength in the hands and fingers, making it easier to perform tasks such as sewing and picking up coins.

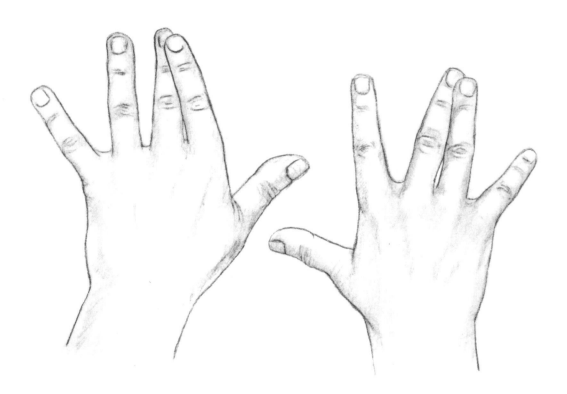

INSTRUCTIONS

1. With open hands, wiggle your fingers in all directions. You may choose to wiggle all your fingers together or each one separately.

2. Continue this motion up to thirty seconds.

Hand Stretch

STARTING POSITION: Standing

DESIRED RESULT: Increased flexibility of the hands and fingers, which improves their range of motion and helps reduce pain.

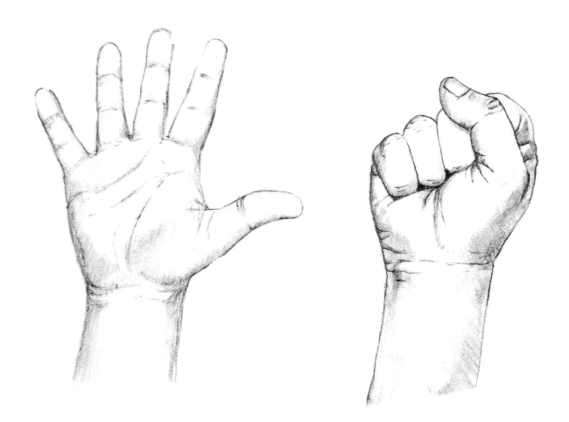

INSTRUCTIONS

1. Open your hands and stretch your fingers until you can feel a pull in the palms of your hands.

2. Make a fist.

3. Repeat up to ten times.

> **If you have arthritis in your hands, move slowly and emphasize the stretching part of this exercise.**

Thumb Stretch

STARTING POSITION: Standing

DESIRED RESULT: Increased flexibility of the hands and thumbs, which improves their range of motion and helps reduce pain.

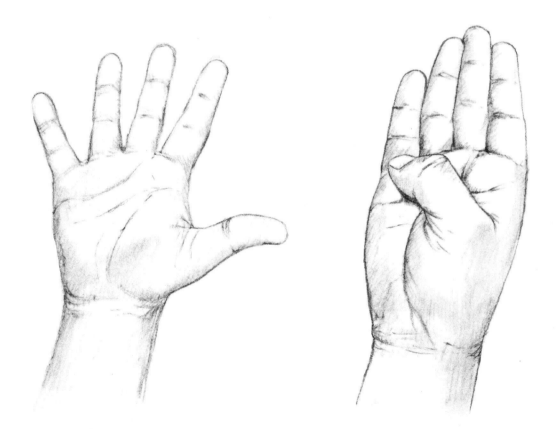

INSTRUCTIONS

1. With your fingers together, bring your thumb across the palm of your hand until it touches the base of your small finger.
2. Return the thumb to the starting position and stretch all your fingers for ten counts.
3. Repeat up to ten times. (You can perform this exercise with both hands at the same time.)

Small-Finger Stretch

STARTING POSITION: Standing

DESIRED RESULT: Increased flexibility of the hands and small fingers, which improves their range of motion and helps reduce pain.

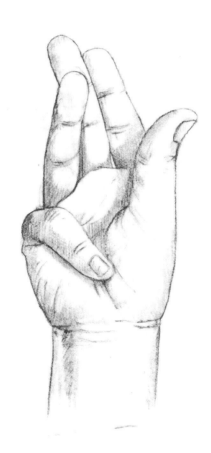

INSTRUCTIONS

1. With your fingers together, bring your small finger across the palm of your hand until it touches the base of your thumb.
2. Return your small finger to the starting position and stretch all your fingers for ten counts.
3. Repeat up to ten times. (You can perform this exercise with both hands at the same time.)

Middle-Finger Stretch 1

STARTING POSITION: Standing

DESIRED RESULT: Increased flexibility of the hands and middle fingers, which improves their coordination. This helps when performing such tasks as handwriting and sewing.

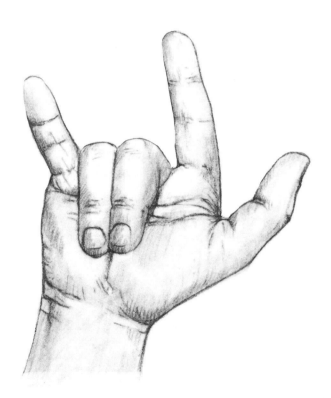

INSTRUCTIONS

1. With fingers extended straight out, bring your two middle fingers down to touch the palm of your hand. The two outside fingers should remain straight up.

2. Return your middle fingers to the starting position, then stretch all fingers for up to ten counts.

3. Repeat up to ten times. (You can do both hands at the same time.)

Middle-Finger Stretch 2

STARTING POSITION: Standing

DESIRED RESULT: Increased flexibility of the hands and middle fingers, which improves their coordination. This helps when performing such tasks as handwriting and sewing.

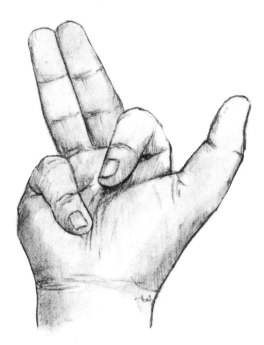

INSTRUCTIONS

1. With your fingers extended straight out, bring your two outside fingers down to touch the palm of your hand. The two inside fingers should remain straight up.

2. Return the outside fingers to the starting position, then stretch all the fingers for up to ten counts.

3. Repeat up to ten times. (You can do both hands at the same time.)

> If you haven't done finger or hand exercises, you may find that your fingers don't like parting from one another. Don't worry, you can develop the coordination to move your fingers—both together and separately—with practice.

Alternating Finger Stretch

STARTING POSITION: Standing

DESIRED RESULT: Increased coordination, strength, and flexibility of the hands and fingers. This helps when performing fine motor-coordination tasks such as handwriting and picking up coins.

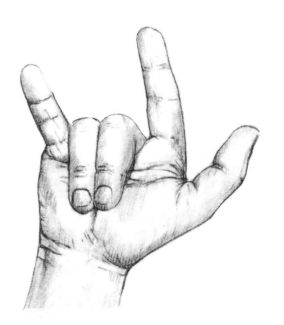 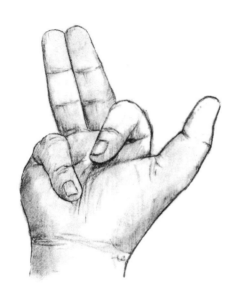

INSTRUCTIONS

1. Keeping your outside fingers up, bring your two middle fingers down to touch the palm of your hand.
2. Then switch, putting your outside fingers down and middle fingers up.
3. Alternate this motion as fast as you can up to ten times. (You can do both hands at the same time.)

Random Wrist Motions

STARTING POSITION: Standing

DESIRED RESULT: Increased range of motion in the wrists, which improves mobility and helps reduce pain.

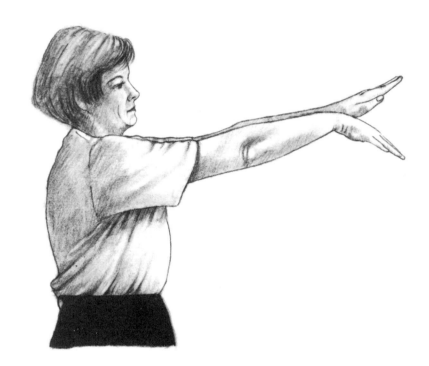

INSTRUCTIONS

1. With arms extended straight out in front of you, bend your hands at the wrists.
2. Move your wrists in all directions while keeping your fingers straight.
3. Repeat up to ten times in all directions.

Wrist Circling

STARTING POSITION: Standing

DESIRED RESULT: Increased range of motion in the wrists, which improves mobility and helps reduce pain.

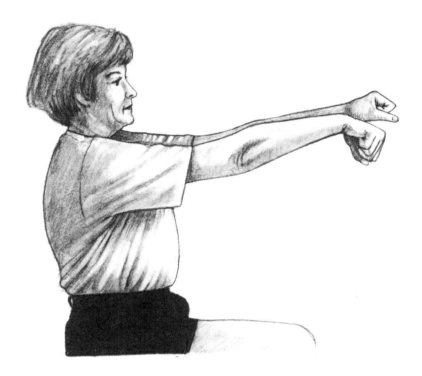

INSTRUCTIONS

1. Circle your wrists up to ten times in one direction and then the other.

2. Repeat up to ten times in each direction.

Exercises for the Torso, Upper Back, and Chest

As we age, our rib cage loses some of its flexibility. Torso exercises increase the flexibility of the muscles in the chest and at the sides of the body. This added flexibility makes breathing easier, improves posture, and allows turning and twisting without back injury. Exercises for the upper back and chest will help improve posture. When muscles tug and pull on bones, the bones become stronger. To prevent osteoporosis, exercises that work on the bones of the upper back are important.

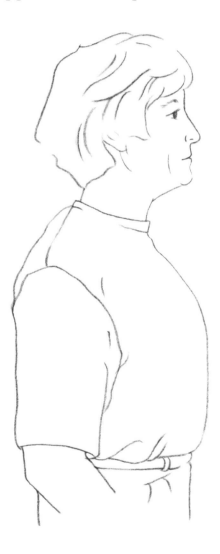

Bent-Arm Raises

STARTING POSITION: Standing

DESIRED RESULT: Increased strength and flexibility of the upper back and chest, which promote good posture.

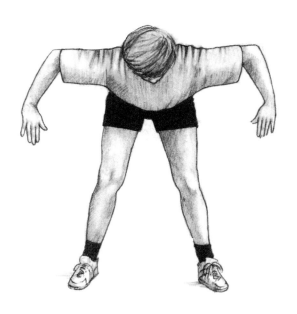 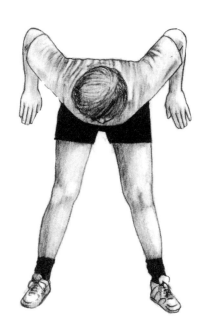

INSTRUCTIONS

1. While bent over at the waist, bend your elbows and raise your arms out to the sides. Your shoulder blades should come together.

2. Repeat up to ten times.

Overhead-Arm and Torso Stretch

STARTING POSITION: Standing

DESIRED RESULT: Increased flexibility of the arms, shoulders, and rib cage, which encourages good posture. Improved rib cage flexibility may also improve breathing.

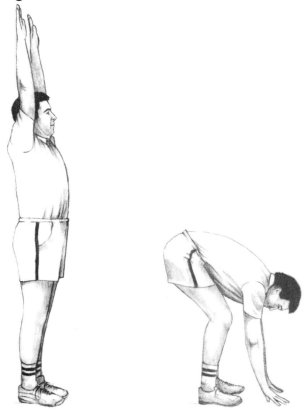

INSTRUCTIONS

1. Reach overhead with outstretched arms.
2. Pull your upper arms in so that they touch the sides of your head.
3. Clasp hands together and pull your arms up. (You'll feel a lifting in the shoulders, ribs, and waist.) While holding this position, take a deep breath and count to ten.
4. Exhale for ten counts while bending down and bringing your arms down to the floor.
5. Inhale and return to the starting position.
6. Repeat up to ten times.

Side Stretch

STARTING POSITION: Standing

DESIRED RESULT: Increased strength and flexibility of the rib cage, and improved strength in the muscles found at the sides of your body. This helps improve breathing and promotes good posture.

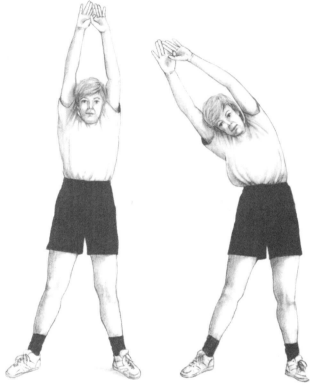

INSTRUCTIONS

1. While standing up straight, inhale and silently count to ten while raising your arms over your head.
2. Exhale for ten counts while leaning to one side.
3. Hold that position for ten counts.
4. Return to the original position.
5. Repeat up to ten times on each side.

> As we age, our rib cage loses some of its flexibility. A rigid rib cage does not allow the lungs to fully inflate. This exercise helps increase the flexibility of the rib cage to make breathing easier.

Exercises for the Abdomen

Strong abdominal muscles are a must for good posture, for keeping the abdominal organs in their proper positions, and for preventing or alleviating lower-back problems. These muscles are generally weak and may take a long time to improve. Be positive. Keep going. Every time you exercise, you are strengthening these muscles. Be careful not to jerk or strain.

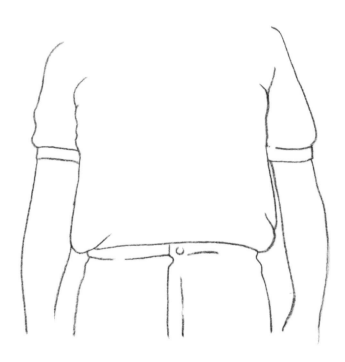

Leg Lowering

STARTING POSITION: Lying on your back (on mat)

DESIRED RESULT: Increased strength in the lower back and abdomen, which helps reduce the chance of back injury and encourages good posture.

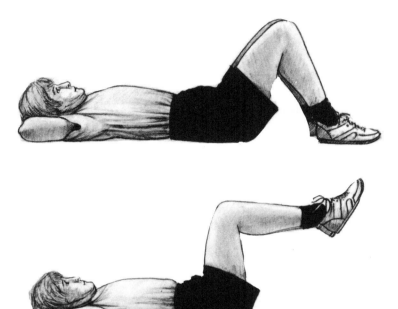

INSTRUCTIONS

1.   Lie on your back with your hands clasped behind your head.
2.   Bend your legs and lift them until your lower legs are parallel to the floor.
3.   Press your lower back against the mat and slowly count to five, lowering your feet to the floor with your knees bent.
4.   Finish with your knees bent and feet flat on the floor.
5.   Repeat up to ten times.

In order to prevent back injuries, it is important to keep your back flat against the floor while lowering your feet. Place a small pillow under the small of your back for added safety.

Leg Extenders

STARTING POSITION: Lying on your back (on mat)

DESIRED RESULT: Increased strength in the lower back and abdomen, which helps reduce the chance of back injury and encourages good posture.

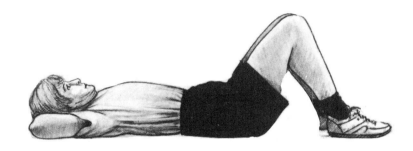

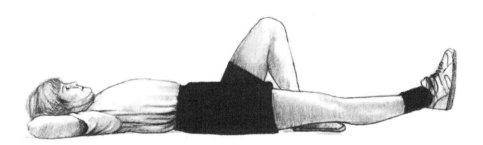

INSTRUCTIONS

1. Lie on your back with your knees bent and your hands clasped behind your head. Keep your lower back against the mat.
2. Extend your right leg until it is completely straight and as close to the floor as possible. (Make sure that your left leg is bent.) Hold this position up to ten counts without holding your breath.
3. Repeat up to ten times with each leg.

To prevent back injuries, make sure one leg stays in the bent position. Make sure you breathe during this exercise. Holding your breath could increase your blood pressure.

Shoulder Raises

STARTING POSITION: Lying on your back (on mat)

DESIRED RESULT: Increased strength of the abdominal muscles, which encourages good posture and helps reduce the chance of back injury.

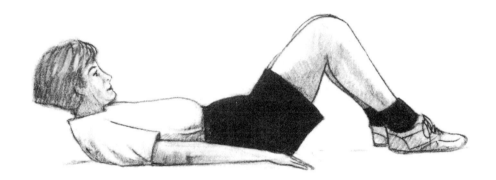

INSTRUCTIONS

1. While lying on your back with knees bent, place your hands at your sides and raise your chin to your chest.
2. Keeping your knees bent and feet flat on the floor, lift your head and shoulders off the floor about twelve inches.
3. Repeat up to ten times.

Make sure you breathe during this exercise. Holding your breath could increase your blood pressure. Exhale as you lift your head and shoulders off the floor.

Leg and Shoulder Raises

STARTING POSITION: Lying on your back (on mat)

DESIRED RESULT: Increased strength in the abdominal muscles, which encourages good posture and reduces the chance of back injury.

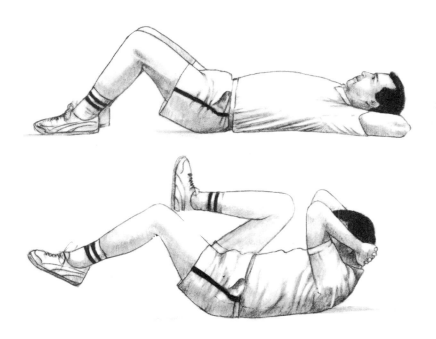

INSTRUCTIONS

1. Lie on your back with your hands clasped behind your head. Bend your knees, keeping your feet flat on the floor.
2. Put your left heel on your right knee.
3. Lift your head, shoulders, foot, and buttocks off the floor at the same time. Attempt to touch your forehead to your left knee.
4. Repeat up to ten times with each leg.

Sit-Backs

STARTING POSITION: Sitting on a mat

DESIRED RESULT: Increased strength in the abdominal muscles, which encourages good posture and reduces the chance of back injury.

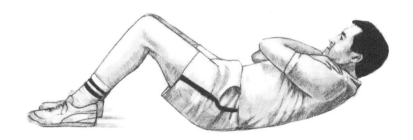

INSTRUCTIONS

1. Sit on the mat with your knees bent and your feet flat on the floor. Cross your arms over your chest.
2. Lean back as far as you can without touching the mat.
3. Return to the upright position without using your hands.
4. Repeat up to ten times.

Make sure you breathe during this exercise. Holding your breath could increase your blood pressure. Exhale as you lift your body back to the sitting position.

Sit-Ups

STARTING POSITION: Sitting on a mat

DESIRED RESULT: Increased strength in the abdominal muscles, which encourages good posture and reduces the chance of back injury.

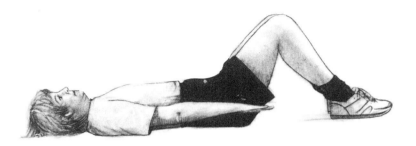

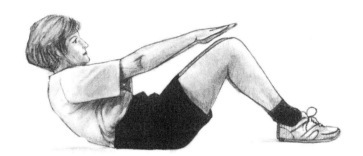

INSTRUCTIONS

1. Sitting with your knees bent and your feet flat on the floor, place your hands straight out in front of you.
2. Lower your torso back until your head and shoulders touch the floor.
3. Exhale and sit up as high as you can.
4. Repeat up to ten times.

- **If you want to maximize the strength in the abdominal muscles, do not use your hands or arms to help you sit up.**

- **Come up only as high as is comfortable. With practice, you will eventually be able to sit up without assistance.**

Exercises for the Hips and Legs

If a quality life is what you desire, you must be independent in doing things for yourself. You must be able to walk, climb stairs, bend down, get up, and do a certain amount of lifting. All of these moves are dependent on strong leg and hip muscles. Having strong, flexible hips will enable you to take longer steps and walk faster, which may help prevent falling. Putting force on the hips also helps increase the strength of the hip bones.

One of the best ways to improve hip and leg muscles is by doing a lot of walking. Muscles respond to stress. If you have trouble walking, then walking is exactly what you should do to improve the situation. The following exercises are excellent examples of hip and leg strengtheners.

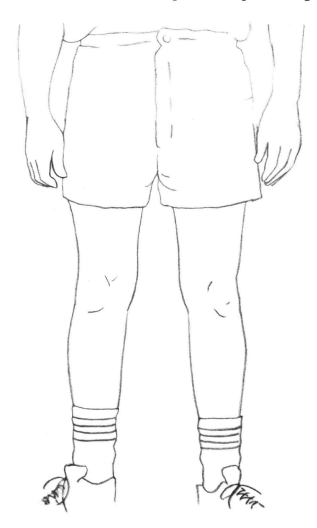

Bottom Raises

STARTING POSITION: Standing

DESIRED RESULT: Increased strength in the upper legs. This helps when performing such movements as getting out of the back seat of a car or a deep chair, and getting up off the floor.

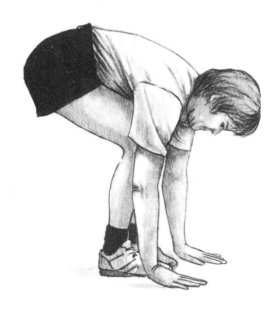

INSTRUCTIONS

1. Squat down so your knees are bent and your palms are flat on the floor.
2. Straighten your legs, keeping a slight bend in the knees to protect your back.
3. Return to the starting position.
4. Repeat up to ten times.

Leg Stretch

STARTING POSITION: Standing

DESIRED RESULT: Increased flexibility of the legs and knees, which makes walking easier.

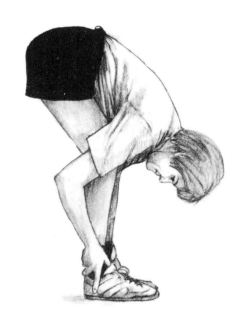

INSTRUCTIONS

1. Stand with your legs together and knees slightly bent. Lean over and grab your ankles with both hands.
2. Pull your chest as close to your thighs as possible. Straighten your legs as much as you can.
3. Hold this position up to thirty seconds.
4. Do this exercise one time.

Calf Stretch

STARTING POSITION: Standing

DESIRED RESULT: Increased flexibility of the lower legs, which makes walking easier.

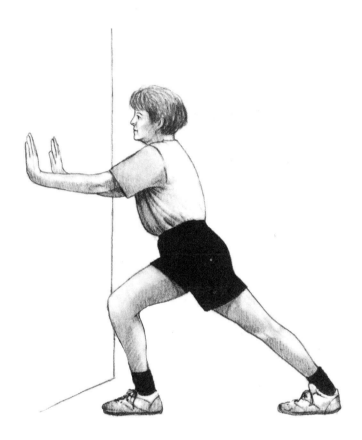

INSTRUCTIONS

1. Straighten your arms in front of you and place both palms (shoulder high) against a wall.
2. Bend your right knee and place your left foot behind you, heel flat on the floor. Keep your left foot pointing straight ahead.
3. Lean into the wall and feel the stretch in your calf and heel.
4. Hold up to thirty seconds.
5. Do this stretch one time with each leg.

Heel Raises

STARTING POSITION: Standing

DESIRED RESULT: Increased strength in the ankles and lower leg. This helps maintain good balance, which reduces the chance of falling.

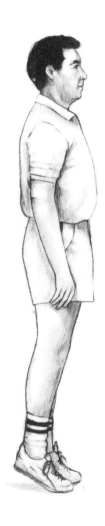

INSTRUCTIONS

1. Stand with your feet flat on the floor and your arms at your sides.

2. Lift your heels off the floor, then return to the starting position.

3. Repeat up to ten times.

Toe Raises

STARTING POSITION: Standing

DESIRED RESULT: Increased strength in the ankles and lower leg. This helps maintain good balance, which reduces the chance of falling.

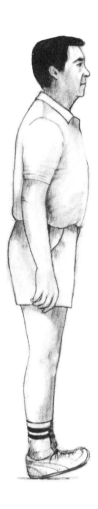

INSTRUCTIONS

1. Stand with your feet flat on the floor and your arms at your sides.

2. Lift your toes off the floor then return to the starting position.
3. Repeat up to ten times.

Leg Raises 1

STARTING POSITION: Lying on your side (on mat)

DESIRED RESULT: Increased strength in the upper-leg and hip muscles, which helps maintain good balance and makes walking easier.

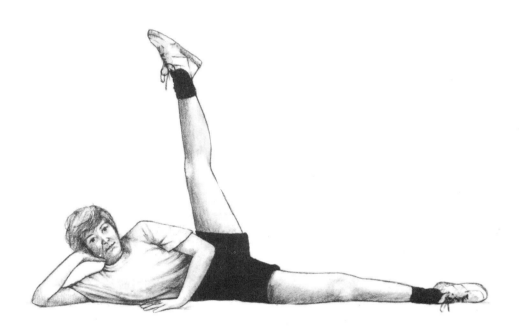

INSTRUCTIONS

1. Lie on your left side while resting on your elbow. Place your right leg on top of your left leg.
2. Raise your right leg as high as you can, then lower it back to the starting position.
3. Repeat up to ten times on each side.

Leg Raises 2

STARTING POSITION: Lying on your side (on mat)

DESIRED RESULT: Increased strength in the upper- leg and hip muscles, which helps maintain good balance and makes walking easier.

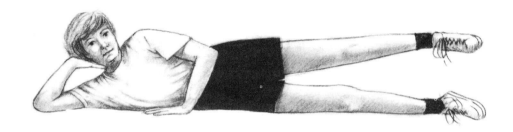

INSTRUCTIONS

1. Lie on your left side while resting on your elbow. Place your right leg on top of your left leg.
2. Raise your right leg about twelve inches. Slowly, to the count of five, return to the starting position.
3. Repeat up to ten times on each side.

Leg Holds

STARTING POSITION: Lying on your side (on mat)

DESIRED RESULT: Increased strength of the upper-leg and hip muscles, which helps maintain good balance and makes walking easier.

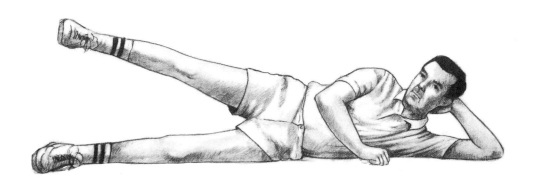

INSTRUCTIONS

1. Lie on your left side while resting on your elbow. Place your right leg on top of your left leg.
2. Raise your right leg about twelve inches and hold this position for ten counts. Return to the starting position.
3. Repeat up to ten times on each side.

Inner-Thigh Raises

STARTING POSITION: Lying on your side (on mat)

DESIRED RESULT: Increased strength in the upper-leg and hip muscles, which helps maintain good balance and makes walking easier.

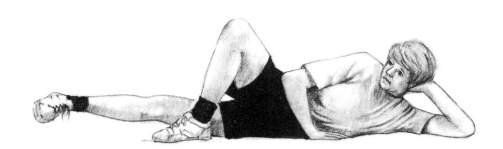

INSTRUCTIONS

1. Lie on your left side while resting on your elbow. Bend your right leg and place your right foot flat on the floor in front of your extended left leg.
2. Lift your left leg off the floor. (Do not rotate your left leg while lifting.) You should feel your inner thigh tightening as you lift.
3. Return to the starting position.
4. Repeat up to ten times on each side.

Leg Lifts

STARTING POSITION: On hands and knees (on mat)

DESIRED RESULT: Increased strength in the upper-leg, hip, and buttock muscles, which helps maintain good balance and makes walking easier.

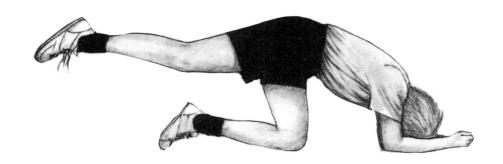

INSTRUCTIONS

1. Get down on your hands and knees. Lower yourself onto your elbows keeping your head down. (This will take the strain off your lower back and neck.)

2. Lift your right leg until it is even with your hip. Keeping this leg straight, lift it as high as you can.

3. Return leg to the hip-high position.

4. Repeat up to ten times with each leg.

Knee-to-Chest Lift

STARTING POSITION: On hands and knees (on mat)

DESIRED RESULT: Increased strength in the upper-leg, hip, and buttock muscles, which helps maintain good balance and makes walking easier.

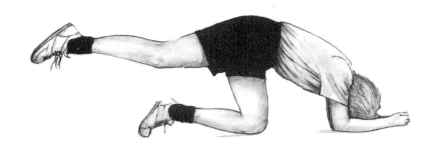

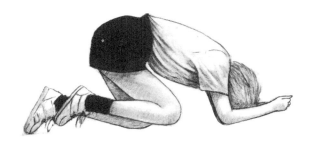

INSTRUCTIONS

1. Get down on your hands and knees. Lower yourself onto your elbows keeping your head down. (This will take the strain off your lower back and neck.)
2. Lift your right leg until it is even with your hip. Bend your right knee and bring it to your chest.
3. Return leg to the hip-high position.
4. Repeat up to ten times with each leg.

Exercises for the Feet and Ankles

We depend on our feet to get us around, but they are often ignored unless we feel pain or discomfort when walking. Foot exercises may seem odd at first, but they are an important part of foot care. These exercises strengthen the toes and feet promoting good balance.

Characteristically, diabetics have poor circulation in the lower extremities. Therefore, good foot care is especially important for those with diabetes.

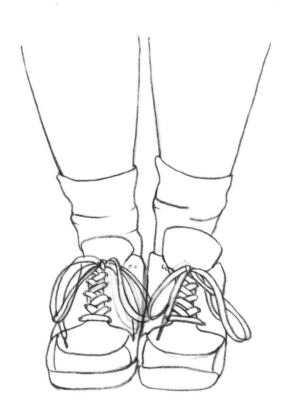

Toe Wiggling

STARTING POSITION: Sitting on a mat

DESIRED RESULT: Increased flexibility of the toes and feet, which promotes good balance.

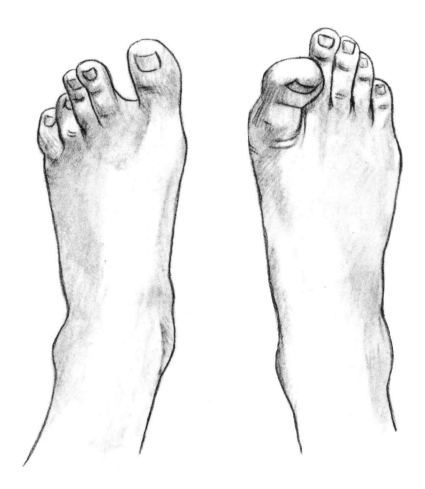

INSTRUCTIONS

1. Remove your shoes and wiggle your toes.

2. Do this up to thirty seconds.

Toe Stretches

STARTING POSITION: Sitting on a mat

DESIRED RESULT: Increased flexibility of the toes and feet, which promotes good balance.

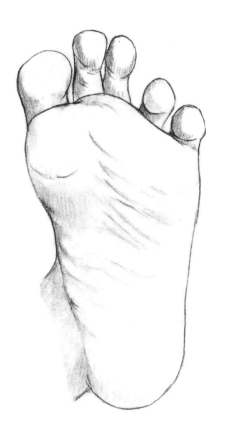 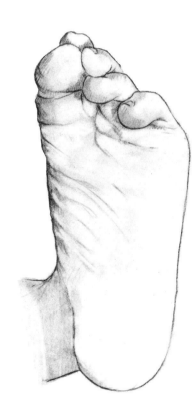

INSTRUCTIONS

1. Remove your shoes and stretch your toes as far apart as you can.
2. Relax the stretch and curl your toes under.
3. Continue stretching and curling up to ten times. (You can perform this exercise with both feet at the same time.)

Toe Lifts

STARTING POSITION: Standing

DESIRED RESULT: Increased strength and flexibility of the feet, which promotes good balance.

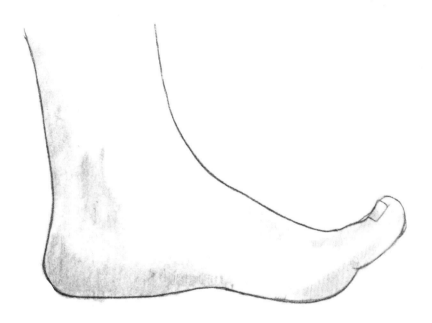

INSTRUCTIONS

1. Remove your shoes and put your feet flat on the floor.
2. Keep the soles of your feet on the floor, and lift all your toes as high as you can.
3. Do this up to ten times. (You can do this exercise with both feet at the same time.)

Big-Toe Lifts

STARTING POSITION: Standing

DESIRED RESULT: Increased strength and flexibility of the big toes, which promote good balance.

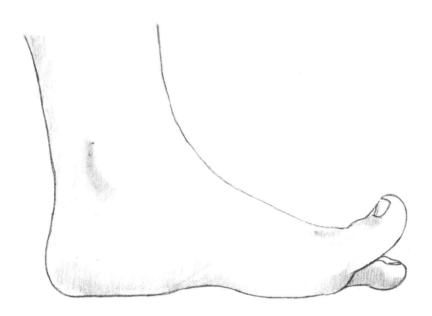

INSTRUCTIONS

1. Remove your shoes and put your feet flat on the floor.
2. Keep the soles of your feet on the floor, and lift up your big toe only.
3. Do this up to ten times. (You can perform this exercise with both feet at the same time.)

If you have a problem lifting your big toe only, hold the small toes down with your fingers.

Small-Toe Lifts

STARTING POSITION: Standing

DESIRED RESULT: Increased strength and flexibility of the feet and toes, which promotes good balance.

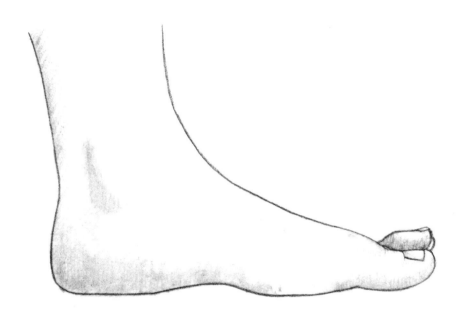

INSTRUCTIONS

1. Remove your shoes and put your feet flat on the floor.
2. Keep the soles of your feet on the floor, and lift your small toes only.
3. Do this up to ten times. (You can perform this exercise with both feet at the same time.)

If you have a problem lifting your small toes only, hold the big toe down with your fingers.

Foot Lifts

STARTING POSITION: Standing

DESIRED RESULT: Increased muscle strength in the lower legs and ankles, which promotes good balance.

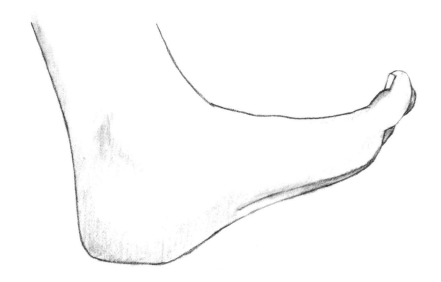

INSTRUCTIONS

1. Remove your shoes and put your feet flat on the floor.
2. Keeping your heels on the floor, lift up the soles of your feet.
3. Repeat up to ten times.

Ankle Rolls

STARTING POSITION: Standing

DESIRED RESULT: Increased strength and flexibility of the feet, which promotes good balance.

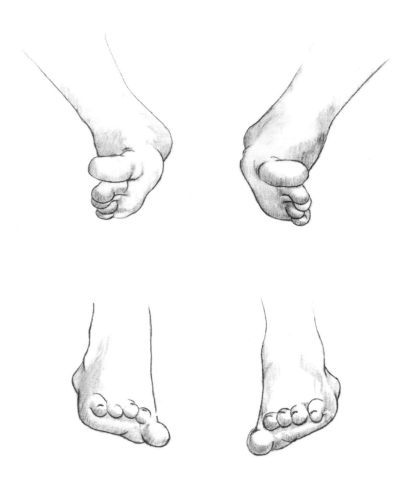

INSTRUCTIONS

1. Roll your feet to the inside edges   2.   Repeat up to ten times.
    and then to the outside edges.

CHAPTER 8
Stretching Exercises

When the connective tissue (tendons, ligaments, and muscles), which surrounds the body's joints, is tight, even simple movements can cause pain. For example, if the connective tissue in the hip area is not flexible, the legs can no longer take long strides, and walking can be reduced to a shuffle. When walking speed slows, the chances of falling increase. A tight, shortened abdominal muscle can interfere with the simple act of standing up straight. This stooped posture can result in digestive, as well as lower-back problems. Keeping this muscle. stretched and flexible helps reduce pain, prevent injury, and improve range of motion.

The following stretching exercises help maintain flexibility in the connective tissue. These exercises can be done alone or in conjuction with the exercises presented in the Sit-Down Workout or in the General Conditioning Workout (Chapters 6 and 7). For your comfort and safety make sure to use a mat when doing the stretching exercises.

Overhead Torso Stretch

STARTING POSITION: Lying on your back (on mat)

DESIRED RESULT: Increased flexibility of the arms, shoulders, torso, and legs, which promotes better movement with less pain.

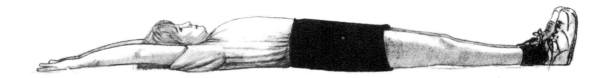

INSTRUCTIONS

1. While lying on your back, stretch your arms overhead.
2. Pull your arms toward your head until they are covering your ears. Press your back and knees a-gainst the mat.
3. Hold this stretched position up to thirty seconds.
4. Do this stretch one time.

Lower-Back Stretch

STARTING POSITION: Lying on your back (on mat)

DESIRED RESULT: Increased flexibility of the lower back, which encourages good posture and reduces the chance of back injury.

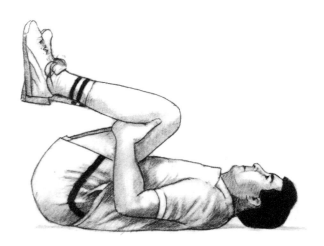

INSTRUCTIONS

1. Lie on your back with your knees bent. Place your hands under your thighs.
2. Pull your thighs toward your chest. You will feel the stretch in your lower back.
3. Hold this stretched position up to thirty seconds.
4. Do this stretch one time.

Alternate Hip Stretch

STARTING POSITION: Lying on your back (on mat)

DESIRED RESULTS: Increased flexibility of the hips, which makes walking easier.

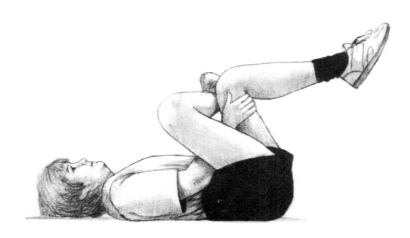

INSTRUCTIONS

1. Lie on your back with your legs extended.
2. Bend your right knee and bring your right foot across your torso and over your left hip. Gently pull your ankle in toward your waist.
3. Bend your left knee and press it against your right foot. Clasp your left knee and pull it toward your left hip. You will feel the stretch in your right hip.
4. Hold this stretched position up to thirty seconds.
5. Do this stretch one time on each side.

Straight-Leg Stretch

STARTING POSITION: Sitting on a mat

DESIRED RESULTS: Increased flexibility of the legs and lower back, which reduces the chance of injury to the lower back.

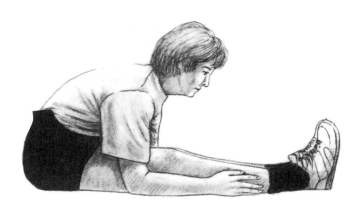

INSTRUCTIONS

1. Sit up with your legs together and extended straight out in front of you. Press your knees to the floor.
2. Lean over and hold on to your legs. Pull your torso as close to your thighs as possible.
3. Hold this stretched position up to thirty seconds.
4. Do this stretch one time.

> **It is not necessary to touch your toes. The important thing is to keep your knees straight when leaning forward. You can judge your progress by watching how your hands move closer to your toes as your flexibility improves.**

Side-Straddle Stretch

STARTING POSITION: Sitting on a mat

DESIRED RESULT: Increased flexibility of the hips, legs, and lower back, which makes walking easier and reduces the chance of injury to the lower back.

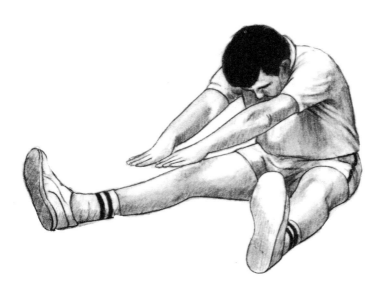

INSTRUCTIONS

1. Sit up with your legs extended straight out in front of you and as far apart as possible. Keep your knees against the floor.
2. Lean forward and stretch your arms out in front of you. You will feel the stretch in your inner thighs, hips, and lower back.
3. Hold this stretched position up to thirty seconds.
4. Do this stretch one time.

Soles-Together Stretch

STARTING POSITION: Sitting on a mat

DESIRED RESULT: Increased flexibility of the hips, legs, and lower back, which makes walking easier and reduces the chance of injury.

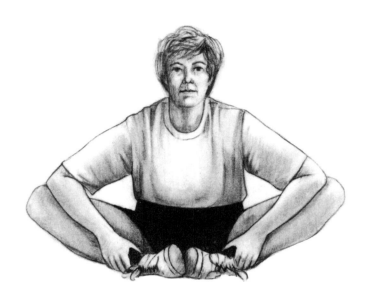

INSTRUCTIONS

1. Sit on the mat with your knees bent and your feet flat on the floor.
2. Drop both knees apart and out to the sides, bringing the soles of your feet together. Pull your heels as close to your body as you can.
3. Hold on to your feet and pull your torso as close to your legs as you can. Push your knees down toward the floor with your elbows. You will feel the stretch in your inner thighs, hips, and lower back.
4. Hold this stretched position up to thirty seconds.
5. Do this exercise one time.

Torso Twister

STARTING POSITION: Sitting on a mat

DESIRED RESULT: Increased flexibility of the torso, which helps reduce the chance of lower-back injury.

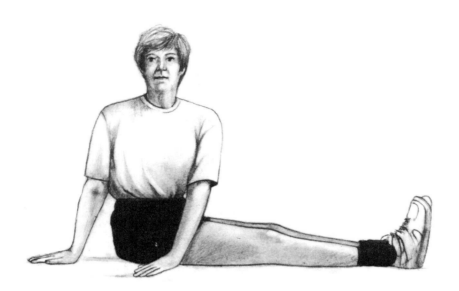

INSTRUCTIONS

1. Sit on the floor with your legs extended straight out in front of you. Straighten your back.
2. Twist to the right, placing both hands flat on the floor to the right of your hip. You will feel the stretch in your torso.
3. Hold this stretch up to thirty seconds.
4. Do this stretch one time on each side.

Toes In-and-Out

STARTING POSITION: Standing

DESIRED RESULT: Increased flexibility of the hips, knees, and ankles, which makes walking easier and reduces the chance of injury.

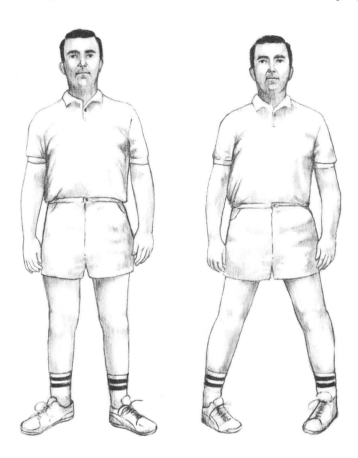

INSTRUCTIONS

1. Stand up keeping both legs straight. Turn your feet inward as far as you can.
2. Hold this stretched position up to thirty seconds.
3. Turn both feet out as far as you can.
4. Hold this stretched position up to thirty seconds. You will feel the stretch in your hips, knees, and ankles.
5. Do this stretch one time.

Rib and Waist Stretch

STARTING POSITION: Standing

DESIRED RESULT: Increased flexibility of the arms, shoulders, and rib cage, which promotes good posture.

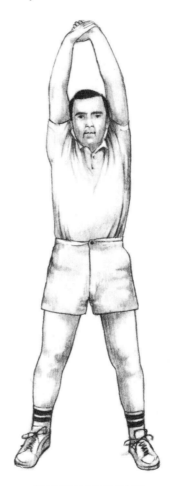

INSTRUCTIONS

1. Stand up straight and stretch your arms overhead, so that your upper arms touch the sides of your head.

2. Clasp your hands together and pull your arms up. You'll feel the stretch in your shoulders, ribs, and waist.

3. Hold the stretch up to thirty seconds.

4. Do this stretch one time.

Upper-Body Stretch

STARTING POSITION: Standing

DESIRED RESULT: Increased strength and flexibility of the rib cage and the sides of your body. This helps improve breathing and promotes good posture.

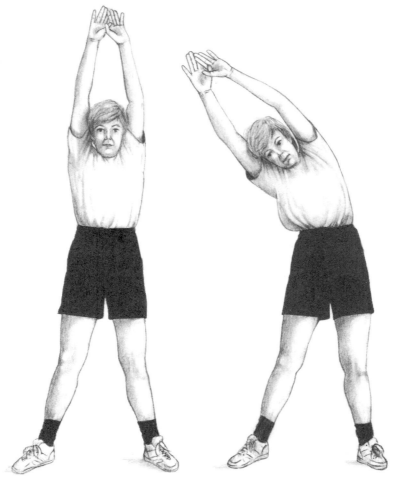

INSTRUCTIONS

1. Stand up straight and stretch your arms overhead, keeping them close to your ears.
2. Keeping your back straight, lean to one side. You will feel a stretch in the side of your body.
3. Hold this stretch up to thirty seconds.
4. Do this exercise one time on each side.

The Evidence Grows

This book describes how older adults can start exercising. Many of you may still be asking yourselves, "Why bother?" Perhaps the most important reason is that the human body is designed to be physically active. When we do not exercise routinely, the inactivity contributes to multiple problems including certain diseases and progressive physical dependency on others (Siebens, 1990).

How do we know our bodies were meant to be physically active? Recent anthropological studies indicate that our ancestors routinely had to have strength and endurance to survive day-to-day as hunters and gatherers (Eaton et al, 1988). For example, after a successful hunt, men, whose average height was 5 feet 2 inches, weighing an average of 112 pounds, would carry forty-five to seventy pounds of fresh meat at three miles an hour over fifteen miles a day. Women, whose average height was 4 feet 11 inches, weighing an average of 93 pounds, would walk two to twelve miles, round trip, to gather food two to three times a week. Clearly, our current lifestyle is significantly more sedentary than this. The most sedentary people in our society are the elderly. In one study of persons twenty to thirty-four years old, 15 percent of the women and 48 percent of the men remained physically active. In those over age fifty, only 1 percent of women and 10 percent of men exercised routinely (Haskell, 1980). The United States Public Health Service Survey reported that less than 20 percent of adults in the United States engage in an amount of exercise sufficient to enhance their cardiovascular status (Stephens et al, 1985).

While we are clearly sedentary, our genes have not changed from those of our ancestors, and evidence is accumulating that demonstrates how our inactive lifestyles are harmful to our health. For example, scientists once thought that the weakness and lack of physical endurance seen in older people was caused by aging and the diseases associated with the aging process. However, numerous exercise studies performed in persons over the age of seventy have shown that muscles can be strengthened 150 percent, and the endurance for continuous exercise can increase 100 percent (Fiatarone,1990). In a three-year study evaluating the effects of an exercise program in women seventy years of age and older, the exercise participants showed improvement in their balance, flexibility, and reaction time. The non-exercisers declined in these skills (Rikli & Edwards, 1991).

These types of studies proved that aging and disease alone do not cause physical deterioration of the elderly. A sedentary lifestyle is the major contributor to physical deterioration. This helps explain the huge variation in physical fitness that is seen in older people. Some seventy-year-olds are able to participate in the Senior Olympics, while others are not able to get out of the bathtub by themselves.

Healthy exercising, in fact, may be one of the best measures to help older adults remain physically independent and continue living in their own homes. Daily activities like carrying groceries, bending down to pick up objects, and walking across the street before the light changes are all related to being physically fit. These same kinds of activities are necessary for people who desire to live by themselves, rather than in a nursing home or under an attendant's care. To date, the decline in physical functioning appears to accelerate in the seventh decade of life (Cunningham & Paterson, 1990) making it particularly important for adults in this age group to participate in an appropriate exercise regimen.

ATTITUDES TOWARD EXERCISE

A few recent studies have examined the attitudes of older persons toward their bodies and exercise. Some elderly people who are not physically fit feel that they engage in enough physical activity (Sidney & Shepard,1977). Progressive education may, therefore, help older persons better understand the important role of exercise and experience some of its benefits.

In another survey of 413 people, where the average age was seventy-seven years old, routine exercisers felt they were in better physical condition, could lift heavy objects without difficulty, could walk faster, and were more flexible than people who did not participate in regular physical-activity classes. In this group of exercisers, 58 percent had arthritis and 29 percent had orthopedic problems. They, nonetheless, reported that they were more physically active than their non-exercising friends who participated in gardening, recreational games, and community activities (Edwards, unpublished). Of note, as well, was that only 10 percent of the exercisers, compared with 17 percent of the non-exercisers, were hospitalized the year of the study. It appears, therefore, that once a person starts to exercise, he experiences improved perceptions of his own abilities. This is seen in the improved performance of daily activities as well as fewer visits to the hospital.

CARDIOVASCULAR FITNESS AND EXERCISE

Keeping the heart strong and healthy is essential for healthy aging. Cardiovascular fitness is measured by how well the body uses oxygen. Think of the heart as a muscle that needs to be exercised like any other muscle in the body. A strong heart is able to keep blood circulating throughout the body. Since blood carries the oxygen needed to turn food into energy, our energy level is determined by the availability of oxygen to the muscles. The way we use oxygen can determine the rate at which we can play or work.

In one study of older men, it was shown that fitness levels could be improved through exercise by about 15 percent over one year. Even more interesting was the fact that these men could do 150 percent more work before they became fatigued (Cunningham & Paterson, 1990).

Besides helping with healthy aging, exercise might be beneficial in preventing coronary artery disease, the major cause of heart disease in America. Coronary artery disease develops when fatty deposits build up on the inner walls of the blood vessels. If this occurs in the coronary arteries feeding the heart, one or more of these arteries might become blocked, resulting in a heart attack or a stroke. There are many factors that can increase your heart-attack potential. These risk factors include diabetes, obesity, smoking, inactivity, emotional stress, high cholesterol, high blood pressure, and a low amount of high-density lipoproteins (HDLs). Though changing your lifestyle may be difficult, increasing your physical activity contributes to reductions in some risk factors. For example, a walking program could help you lose weight; reduce your stress level, blood pressure, and blood sugar; and increase your HDLs.

Even though it is not possible to say for sure, evidence is certainly suggestive that habitual exercise will result in a slower progression of artery closure. Exercise seems to inhibit the initiation and progression of this disease by reducing blood pressure, lowering cholesterol levels, and increasing the good kind of cholesterol [HDLs] (Wood & Stefanick, 1990). Exercise also lowers the low-density lipoproteins (LDLs) and triglycerides. In addition, exercise leads to reduced platelet stickiness and increased insulin sensitivity, which has a bearing on cardiovascular disease (Patsch, 1983).

Regular physical activity seems to protect against coronary heart disease (CHD) in a variety of ways. The most obvious results of aerobic exercise are a slower heart rate, lower blood pressure, and a more efficient heart, which leads to more blood being pumped with each beat. People who are active and physically fit have larger coronary vessels than those of sedentary, less-fit individuals. Exercise also leads to an increased cardiac output and greater work capacity. (Paffenbarger, 1987).

In Finland, doctors compared the electrocardiograms of physically active lumberjacks with those of men who were desk bound or did little moving about. Physical examinations of those active and less-active groups supported the case for regular exercise. The group of sedentary workers had 75 percent more heart irregularities than the more active lumberjacks (deVries,1974).

Dr. Taylor and his colleagues at the University of Minnesota collected data on the risk factors of heart disease. They discovered that the death rate from heart disease among clerks who sat at their desks was more than twice that of men in more active professions (Taylor, 1962).

All these studies show that the inclusion of regular, moderate exercise makes sense for many reasons. Not only will exercise increase your energy level, it will help reduce your risk of coronary heart disease.

BLOOD PRESSURE AND EXERCISE

Hypertension is often called the silent killer because it usually has no symptoms. It is one of the most serious diseases in America. In this country, many people feel that it is normal for blood pressure to increase with age. If your blood pressure is 160/95 at any age you have three times the risk of developing coronary heart disease and four times the chance of having a stroke (Kannel et al, 1984). How does exercise help reduce blood pressure? Basically, two physiological mechanisms occur. One is the lowering of the resting heart rate, which reduces the resistance in the blood vessels, and second is the dilation of blood vessels, which allows a reduction in pressure.

The results of fifteen epidemiological studies were reviewed (Montoye et al. 1972). It was concluded that when a difference was noted between active and inactive populations, the active group always had the lower blood pressure. It was also noted that the more active group had less body fat. Increased caloric expenditure, which in turn causes a decrease in body weight, may be the reason that blood pressure goes down during regular exercise.

Endurance exercise is the type that helps reduce blood pressure. Aerobic exercise falls into the endurance-exercise category. On the other hand, isometric exercise and weightlifting cause a response that increases blood pressure. In a study by Hagberg (1990), it was shown that in older hypertensives, blood pressure decreased after three months of low-intensity (40 to 60 percent of age-adjusted maximum heart rate—see Chapter 5) aerobic exercise. No one knows just how how long it takes for endurance training to lower blood pressure, but we do know that even a single bout of aerobic exercise will cause a decrease it both systolic and diastolic pressure (Hagberg, 1990).

Most individuals with high blood pressure can lower it by about 10mmHg (millimeters of mercury) on the average with endurance-exercise training. It is also important to lose body weight, which can be the result of a good exercise program. *It is important to consult your physician or health-care provider before engaging in any exercise program to control your blood pressure.*

WEIGHT CONTROL AND EXERCISE

Exercise alone may or may not have a positive effect on losing weight. Many variables determine the success of a weight-loss program. Motivation, the amount of food eaten, the type of food eaten (such as a high-fat diet), the length of time spent exercising, the type of exercises performed, and the number of times you have dieted all play a role in successful weight loss. On the other hand, dieting may or may not have a positive effect on losing weight. Historically, when one goes off a diet, the weight usually returns because a permanent change in lifestyle has not occured.

A weight-loss study was done that included twelve women who were at least 40 percent overweight. These twelve women were divided into three groups. One group exercised, another group dieted, and the third group followed a program that included both diet and exercise. Exercising consisted of walking or bicycling for one hour per day, four days a week for six weeks. The results of the study were as follows: An average of 6.4 pounds was lost by each person in the group that dieted only; in the group that exercised only, each person lost an average of 4 pounds; and in the group that dieted and exercised, each person lost an average of 9.1 pounds (Dudleston et al, 1970).

Calorie-restrictive diets can decrease the important vitamins and minerals that are necessary to maintain good health. Some people mistakenly think an increase in exercise causes an increase in appetite, however, just the opposite is true. A study by Dr. Mayer and colleagues at Harvard University showed that sedentary workers ate more and were heavier than those who were physically active (Mayer, Ray & Mitra, 1956). When one diets, the body goes into an energy-saving mode during which time the metabolic rate decreases. This causes a decrease in the energy cost of a particular task. The combination of the decrease in the resting metabolic rate and the energy cost of tasks may be why we have the plateau effect that occurs during weight-loss diets. It has been suggested that exercise training may increase metabolic rate and maintain the lean body mass. Therefore, by combining exercise with reduced-calorie intake you will lose more body fat (Brownell & Stuckard, 1980).

On the other hand, physical conditioning increases active tissue mass and melts fat (provided the caloric intake remains constant). As one ages, muscle tissue is lost. Muscle tissue is active; it helps burn up the food we eat. Physical activity prevents the loss of muscle tissue and enables food to be burned faster. The immediate effect of exercise related to weight loss is that you burn calories while you exercise. Combined with a calorie-restrictive diet, exercise can help with weight loss or weight control. For example, if you exercise at a moderate level for thirty to forty minutes, four days a week, you could use up approximately 1,000 calories a week. The second bonus of a regular exercise program is that you continue to burn fat for about six hours after you have finished exercising (deVries & Gray, 1963). This, alone, could add up to five pounds a year.

It seems that in order to be successful in losing weight, one must make permanent changes involving exercise and good eating habits. No one says that this is easy. It is important to go slowly when beginning an endurance program designed to lose weight (see Chapter 5 on aerobic exercise). Studies have shown that walking rather than jogging is safer if you are overweight (Bray, 1990). Running can cause musculoskeletal problems with your feet, knees, and lower back. In order to decrease body fat, one has to exercise thirty to forty-five minutes, three to four times a week (Pollack et al, 1975). And don't forget that continued exercise will keep you from gaining more weight.

MENTAL HEALTH AND EXERCISE

It has been well documented that physical activity improves physical health. A person's health is multidimensional; it includes the physical as well as the mental component. It is estimated that 25 percent of the population suffers from mild to moderate depression, anxiety, and other indicators of emotional disorder at any given time. Although most of these people are not classified as mentally ill, they still suffer and seek assistance (Brown, 1990). Many people suffer with these problems but do not seek professional help.

A study conducted by the United States Government showed that physical activity elevated mood, increased feelings of well-being, and reduced anxiety and depression (Stepthens, 1988). High levels of muscular tension are related to adverse psychophysiological problems such as tension headaches. deVries (1974) found that a group of older men and women who exercised for four weeks had less electrical activity in their muscles than a group that did not exercise.

Many other studies suggest that chronic exercise reduces depression. Even though we do not know the mechanism by which the reduction of depression occurs, we do know that individuals who are mildly or moderately depressed and who may be at risk for experiencing more severe forms of clinical depression have benefited from long-term aerobic exercise (Brown, 1990).

I have often heard that as people get older they have trouble sleeping. Aerobically fit athletes tend to sleep longer and have elevated slow-wave sleep patterns when compared to matched sedentary control subjects (Paxton et al, 1983). There have not been any studies done with older people that have measured sleep changes with exercise; however, it stands to reason that if one has less anxiety, is less depressed, and feels better about himself, he will probably sleep better, also.

Even though we know that exercise can help elevate mood, reduce depression, and promote increased feelings of well-being, we have no evidence that exercise can prevent mental illness. Perhaps regular aerobic exercise can be, however, an effective management strategy, which might prevent stress-related emotions from becoming a more serious problem.

ARTHRITIS AND EXERCISE

Osteoarthritis is the most common form of arthritis. National Institute of Health records indicate that nearly everyone over the age of sixty has osteoarthritis. This condition is commonly known as the "wear and tear disease" because of its slow, non-inflammatory, degenerative effect upon joint cartilage. The symptoms usually include increasing pain and stiffness. The management of arthritis involves a multidimensional approach. The main objectives of an exercise program are to relieve pain, maintain and improve joint motion, and delay further joint damage. Athletic training does not cause osteoarthritis, but it could cause injury and joint malalignment. It is, therefore, necessary to emphasize safety while participating in sports and games. Physical activities should never include strong abrupt force on the affected joints because this could cause further damage and pain (Smith et al, 1990). Even though there is no medical cure for arthritis, the proper balance of rest and exercise can restore and maintain functional mobility (Piscopo, 1985). Gentle range-of-motion and stretching exercises (see Chapters 6 and 8) are beneficial if you have osteoarthritis.

OSTEOPOROSIS AND EXERCISE

The loss of bone mass and bone strength is a common problem in the elderly population. This condition is called osteoporosis. Osteoporosis can occur in both men and women, but older women are affected most often. The factors associated with this disease are aging, loss of hormones after menopause, lack of calcium and other vitamins, and a sedentary lifestyle.

Of these risk factors, the maintenance of physical activity seems to be one of the most effective methods of preventing this problem.

If you have not exercised in a long time, it is important that you begin your exercise program slowly. Improving your muscle strength is the most important objective. The force on your bones will be reduced. This lessens your chance of falling, which can lead to bone fractures. Regular exercise improves muscle tone, posture, mobility, balance, strength, and flexibility. All of which lead to steadiness and better balance.

Smith and colleagues studied fifty-one nursing-home women over a three-year period. These researchers found that those who participated in a sit-down chair-exercise program showed an increase of 4.2 percent in their bone mass, whereas the non-exercising women actually lost 2.5 percent (Smith et al, 1981).

Since bone mass is dependent upon stress and force, exercise is an important factor, both as a means to increase bone mass and to prevent further deterioration.

DIABETES AND EXERCISE

Diabetes mellitus can be divided into two types: Type I and Type II. Type I results when an insufficient amount of insulin is produced by the pancreas and the patient must take insulin. For this patient, exercise will not help control his diabetes. However, if he wishes to exercise, it is very important that he works out a program with his doctor or health-care provider.

The Type II diabetic is the patient who has multiple problems (cardiovascular risk, excess weight, over sixty years old) but does not need to take insulin. Maturity-onset diabetes can oftentimes be controlled by good dietary and exercise habits. It is well known that exercise training reduces the risks associated with coronary heart disease and reduces weight, which are both very important considerations for this type diabetic patient.

Shepard believes that activity is a particularly valuable treatment for elderly diabetic patients since as many as 30 percent are unable to understand the simple components of a planned diet (Shepard, 1978). In the non-insulin-dependent diabetic, moderate exercise improves insulin secretion. These effects are independent of weight loss (Trovati et al, 1984). *As with anyone beginning an exercise program, the diabetic must begin slowly and be under the careful supervision of a doctor or health-care provider.*

CANCER AND EXERCISE

There is certainly strong evidence that exercise helps reduce the risks associated with heart disease. That exercise will reduce the chances of getting cancer is a new idea. There is, however, a growing amount of data suggesting that exercise reduces the chance of getting certain types of cancer.

One group of researchers in Southern California studied 2,950 men who had colon cancer (Garabrant et al, 1984). These men were classified as having highly physical, moderately physical, or sedentary jobs. It was found that the men with the sedentary jobs had a threefold increased risk of colon cancer than those with the more active jobs. Similar findings appeared in two other studies.

Women athletes were studied by Frisch et al (1985). The athletes had considerably less incidents of cancer of the uterus, ovaries, cervix, vagina, and breast than the non-athletes.

The lower incidence of colon cancer among active people may be explained by several factors. Exercise increases the transit time of waste material and thus reduces the time that toxic materials can be exposed to the lining of the bowel. Since obesity is one of the factors leading to an increased risk of cancer, regular aerobic exercise reduces body fat and body weight. Exercisers might be more aware of the types of food they eat and, therefore, might stay away from a high-fat diet. On the basis of the available evidence, it is likely that women who exercise when they are young may induce certain hormonal changes (less estrogen production), which act as a protectant to reduce the chances of breast and reproductive-organ cancers.

There is little information about the effects of exercise on the patient with cancer. It is doubtful that exercise can reduce or eliminate tumors, but there is good reason to believe that exercise can improve the quality of life.

EXERCISE AND THE LOWER BACK

Lower-back problems in the United States have increased 2,500 percent in the last twenty years (Nachemson, 1990). This change has not occurred because of lifestyle changes or more hazardous work places. It is postulated that back pain may be caused and prolonged by inactivity.

Early, easy movement on an area of the back is an important part of healing (Nachemson,1990). Endurance-type activities, such as swimming or walking, are recommended for disk and cartilage injuries. It is suggested to begin exercising slowly, gradually working up to thirty minutes per day. The increased circulation in the body is actually more important than strong back muscles.

It is interesting to note that, generally, people who are the least fit are more likely to have lower-back pain. However, there is no evidence that fitness prevents lower-back pain. It seems that weak large-muscle groups, particularly the lower-back extensors, seems to put one at greater risk of experiencing pain. It is apparent that patients with acute and chronic back problems do benefit from good exercise programs that provide increase in strength, flexibility, and endurance.

IN CONCLUSION

The aging process begins at birth. Those who study aging agree that getting older is a continuing process during the whole life span. Exercise is necessary throughout this life span for both mental and physical health. Exercise may also be of value in disease prevention. Fortunately, older adults are beginning to exercise more. Hopefully, this may lead to an overall better quality of life.

References

American Association of Retired Persons. September Bulletin, 1987.

Browell, K.D. and A.J. Stuckard. "Physical Activity in the Development and Control of Obesity," *Obesity.* Philadelphia: W.B. Saunders, 1980.

Brown, R.A., D.E. Rameriz, and J.M. Taub. "The Prescription of Exercise for Depression," *Physician and Sports Medicine,* 1978, vol.6, pp. 34–45.

Cooper, Steve. "Hulda on High," *Walking,* September 1987, p. 35.

Cunningham, D.A. and D.H. Peterson. *Exercise, Fitness, and Health: A Consensus of Current Knowledge,* C. Bouchard, R. Shepard, T. Stephens, J. Sutton, B. McPherson, (Ed.). Illinois: Human Kinetics Books, 1990.

Geist, J.H., M.H. Klein, R.R. Eischens, J. Faris, A.S. Gurman, and W.P. Morgan. "Running as a Treatment for Depression." *Comprehensive Psychiatry,* 1979, vol. 53, pp. 20–41.

deVries, H.A. "Neuromuscular Tension and Its Relief," *Journal of the Association for Physical and Mental Rehabilitation,* 1962, vol. 16, pp. 86–88.

deVries, H.A. *Vigor Regained.* New Jersey: Prentice Hall, 1974.

deVries, H.A. and D.E. Gray. "After Effects of Exercise Upon Resting Metabolic Rate," *Research Quarterly,* 1963, vol. 34, pp. 314–321.

Dienbier, R., J. Geigst, and W. Morgan. "Brighter Days," *Runners World,* November 1986, p. 38.

Dudleston, A.K. and M. Bennion. *Effect of Diet and/or Exercise on Obese College Women.* 1970, vol. 56, pp. 126–129.

Eaton, S.B., M. Shostak, and M. Konner. *The Paleolithic Prescription: A Program of Diet and Exercise and a Design for Living.* New York: Harper and Row, 1988.

Fiatarone M. "90-year-olds Show Gains in Weight-Training Study," *Journal of the American Medical Association. Los Angeles Times*, 13 June 1990, p. A16.

Frisch, R.E., G. Wyshak, T.E. Albright, I. Schiff, K.P. Jones, T. Witsihi, E. Shiang, and E. Koff. "Lower Prevalence of Breast Cancer and Cancers of the Reproductive System Among Former College Athletes Compared to Non-Athletes." *British Journal of Cancer*, 1985, vol. 52, pp. 885–891.

Garabrant, D.H., J.M. Peters, T.M. Mack, and L. Bernstein. "Job Activity and Colon Cancer Risk," *American Journal of Epidemiology*, 1984, vol. 119, pp. 1005–1014.

Hagberg, J.M. "Exercise, Fitness and Hypertension," *Exercise, Fitness, and Health: a Consensus of Current Knowledge*, C. Bouchard, R.Shepard, T. Stephens, J. Sutton, and B. McPherson, (Ed.). Illinois: Human Kinetics Books, 1990.

Hagberg, J.M., S.J. Montain, W.H. Martin, and A.A. Ehsani. "Effect of Exercise Training on 60–69 Year-Old Essential Hypertensives," *Exercise, Fitness, and Health: a Consensus of Current Knowledge*, C. Bouchard, R. Shepard, T. Stephens, J. Sutton, and B. McPherson, (Ed.). Illinois: Human Kinetics Books, 1990.

Haskell, W.L., H.L. Taylor, P.D. Wood, A. Schrot, and G. Heiss. "Strenuous Physical Activity, Treadmill Exercise Test Performance and Plasma High Density Lipoprotein Cholesterol," *Circulation*, 1980, vol. 62, pp. 53–59.

Jacobson, E. "The Course of Relation of Muscles of Athletes," *American Journal of Psychology*, 1936, vol. 48, pp. 98–108.

Jennings, R. "Blood Pressure Readings," *Researcher*, 1964, vol. 5.

Kannel, W.B., J.T. Doyle, A.M. Ostfeld, C.D. Jenkins, L. Kuller, R.N. Podell, and J. Stamler. "Original Resources for Primary Prevention of Atherosclerotic Diseases," *Circulation*, 1984, vol. 70, pp. 137A–205A.

Karpatkin, R.H. (Executive Director), "Exercise and Your Heart," *Consumer Research Magazine*, 15 November 1983.

Kavanaugh, T.R., R.H. Shepard, and V. Pandit. "Marathon Running after Myocardial Infarction," *Journal of American Medical Association*, 1974. vol. 229, pp. 1602–1605

Lamb, D.R. *Physiology of Exercise, Responses and Adaptations*. New York: Macmillan Publishing Co., 1984.

Mayer, J., P. Roy, T. P. Mitra. "Relation between Caloric Intake, Body Weights and Physical Work: Studies in an Industrial Mall Population in West Bengal," *American Journal of Clinical Nutrition*, 1956, vol. 4, pp. 169–175.

Modern Maturity. "A Lifetime Learning Minicourse," August–September, 1989, pp. 60–63.

Montoye, H.J., H.L. Metsner, and J.B. Keffar. "Habitual Physical Activity and Blood Pressure," *Medicine, Science and Sport*, 1972, vol. 4, pp. 175–181.

Morehouse, L. and A. Miller. *Exercise Physiology*, 6 ed. St. Louis: Mosby, Inc., 1971.

Morgan, W.P. "Anxiety Reduction Following Acute Physical Activity," *Psychiatry Annuals*, 1971, vol. 9, pp. 36–45.

Nachemeson, A. L. "Exercise, Fitness and Back Pain," *Exercise, Fitness, and Health: a Consensus of Current Knowledge*, C. Bouchard, R. Shepard, T. Stephens, J. Sutton, and B. McPherson, (Ed.). Illinois: Human Kinetics Books, 1990.

National Council on Aging. *The Myth and Reality of Aging in America*, Washington D.C.: NCOA, 1976.

National Institutes of Health. *National Commission on Arthritis and Related Diseases: The Arthritis Plan*. Vol. 1, DHEW, 1976, no. 76, p. 102.

Paffenbarger, Ralph. "The Health Benefits of Exercise," *The Physican and Sports Medicine*, 1987, vol. 15, no. 10, pp. 115–132.

Patsch, J. "Exercise and Hardy Hearts," *Science Digest*, 1983, vol. 91, p. 25.

Paxton, S.J., J. Trinder, and I. Montgomery. "Does Aerobic Fitness Affect Sleep?" *Psychophysiology*, 1983, vol. 20, pp. 320–324.

Piscopo, J. *Fitness and Aging*. New York: John Wiley & Sons, 1985.

Rikli, R.E. and D.E. Edwards. "Effects of a Three-year Exercise Program on Motor Function and Cognitive Processing Speed in Older Women," *Research Quarterly for Exercise and Sport*, 1991, vol. 62, pp. 61–67.

Selve, H. *The Stress of Life*. New York: McGraw Hill Publishers, 1956.

Shepard, R. A. *Physical Activity and Aging*. Chicago: Year Book Publishers, 1978.

Sidney, K.H., and R.J. Shepard. "Activity Patterns of Elderly Men and Women," *Journal of Gerontology*, 1977, vol. 32, pp. 25–32.

Siebens, H. "Deconditioning," *Geriatric Rehabilitation.* B. Kemp, K. Brummel-Smith, J. Ramsdell, (Ed.). Boston: Little Brown, 1990.

Sinaki, M., and B.A. Mikkelsen. "Postmenopausal Spinal Osteoporosis: Flexion Versus Extension Exercises," *Archives of Physical Medical Rehabilitation*, 1984, vol. 65, pp. 234–236.

Smith, E.L., W. Reddan, and P. E. Smith. "Physical Activity and Calcium Modalities for Bone Mineral Increase in Aged Women." *Medicine and Science in Sport*, 1981, vol. 13, pp. 60–64.

Stevens, T. "Physical Activity and Mental Health in the U.S. and Canada in 1990," *Exercise, Fitness, and Health: a Consensus of Current Knowledge*, C. Bouchard, R. Shepard, T. Stephens, J. Sutton, B. McPherson, (Ed.), Illinois: Human Kinetics Books, 1990.

Stevens, T., D.R. Jacobs, and C. C. White. "A Descriptive Epidemiology of Leisure Time Physical Activity," *Exercise, Fitness, and Health: a Consensus of Current Knowledge*, C. Bouchard, R. Shepard, T. Stephens, J. Sutton, B. McPherson, (Ed.), 1990, Illinois: Human Kinetics Books, 1990.

Taylor, H.L., E. Klepetar, A. Keys, W. Parlin, H. Blackborn, and T. Puchner. "Death Rates Among Physically Active and Sedentary Employees of the Railway Industry," *American Journal of Public Health*, 1962, vol. 52, pp. 1697–1707.

Trovati, M., Q. Carta, F. Cavolot, S. Vitali, C. Banaudi, P. Lucchina, F. Fiocchi, G. Emanuelli, and G. Lenti. "Influences of Physical Training on Blood Glucose Control, Glucose Tolerance, Insulin Secretion, and Insulin Action in Non-insulin Dependent Diabetic Patients," C. Bouchard, R. Shepard, T. Stephens, J. Sutton, and B. McPherson, (Ed.), 1990, Illinois: Human Kinetics Books.

U.S. News and World Report. "If You Live to be 100—It Won't be Unusual," 9 May 1983, p. 53.

Wood, P. "Brighter Days," *Runners World*, November 1986, p. 38.

Wood, P. and M. L. Stefanick. "Exercise, Fitness, and Atherosclerosis," *Exercise, Fitness, and Health: a Consensus of Current Knowledge*, C. Bouchard, R. Shepard, T. Stephens, J. Sutton, B. McPherson, (Ed.), 1990, Illinois: Human Kinetics Books.

Index